DATE DUE

FEB 2 6 2003	

RECONSTRUCTING
ILLNESS

RECONSTRUCTING
ILLNESS

Studies in
Pathography

Anne Hunsaker Hawkins

PURDUE UNIVERSITY PRESS
WEST LAFAYETTE, INDIANA

97 96 95 94 93   5 4 3 2 1

Printed in the United States of America

Design by H. Lind Babcock

Library of Congress Cataloging-in-Publication Data

Hawkins, Anne Hunsaker, 1944–
    Reconstructing illness : studies in pathography / by Anne Hunsaker Hawkins
        p.   cm.
    Includes bibliographical references and index.
    ISBN 1-55753-030-0 (alk. paper). —ISBN 1-55753-038-6 (pbk. : alk. paper)
    1. Sick—United States—Biography—History and criticism. 2. Sick—United States—Psychology. 3. Autobiography. 4. Biography as a literary form. 5. Diseases—United States—Public opinion. I. Title.
    [DNLM: 1. Attitude to Death. 2. Attitude to Health. 3. Autobiography, 4. Disease—psychology. 5. Patients—psychology.
        W 85 H393r]
    R726.5.H38 1993
    362.1'092'273—dc20
    DNLM/DLC   92-49892
    for Library of Congress   CIP

To my father and mother
Robert Lee Mitchell and Mae Brooks Mitchell

CONTENTS

✧

This is a study of the myths, attitudes, and assumptions that inform the way we deal with illness. It begins as an analysis of a popular literary genre—recent autobiographies and biographies that describe experiences of illness—but evolves into a discussion of issues in contemporary medical practice. The changing focus of this study, which moves from the literary to the medical and from myth to praxis, reflects a similar development in the life of its author.

My interest in pathographies began when I was revising my doctoral thesis as a book on conversion in spiritual autobiography. It was while I was studying Calvin's *Institutes* and pondering the intricacies of seventeenth-century spiritual regeneration that my father quite unexpectedly suffered a ruptured cerebral aneurysm. It left him—even after expert surgery—partially paralyzed, severely aphasic, and in some way a different person. He died nine years later, and those intervening years were a time of great difficulty, stress, and pain for both my father and my mother. For me, the events of his illness made the nuances of a seventeenth-century conversion seem remote and irrelevant to the suffering experienced in the "real" world.

It is not surprising that I became interested in the accounts of others' illnesses—accounts that dealt graphically and at first hand with catastrophic illness, the miseries of patienthood, and the problematic impact of advanced medical technology. With special fascination, I read Oliver Sacks's *Awakenings*, zealously looking up the unfamiliar technical terms in the glossary provided at the end of the book in order to understand the strange phenomena he describes with such empathy and such meticulous scientific precision. The very title of his book resonated with those spiritual awakenings I had been researching. I began to wonder if there were not some congruence—even some hidden continuity—between these older paradigms of religious sickness and healing and the patterns of experiencing illness and recovery today. I wondered, too, if contemporary pathographies, like the spiritual autobiographies I studied, revealed significant truths about the cultures and value systems from which they sprang. Since I am a scholar, it was inevitable that the attempt to answer such questions took the form of critical essays and addresses. I began to publish in such journals as *Literature and Medicine* and the *Journal of Medicine and Philosophy* and to give talks at meetings of the Society for Health and Human Values. But I still thought of myself as a literary scholar studying literary works in the conventional literary ways.

In 1990, a position opened in the Humanities Department at the Pennsylvania State University College of Medicine. I applied for it and was appointed. Thus for the last two years, I have found myself teaching literature to medical students in a tertiary care medical center. For me, the change is, if not a conversion, certainly an awakening. I am confronted by a new challenge: my students, as well as my medical colleagues, want to know the relevance of literature to their professional work and their professional lives. In addition to modern pathographies and "doctor stories," I teach ancient classics such as Dante's *Inferno* and Sophocles' Oedipus plays. Besides their obvious literary and cultural value, I see an analogous relevance in these great texts to crucial issues in medical practice. These books are not only true and beautiful and good: they are—or can be— useful because they provide paradigms for experience that are surprisingly relevant to the medical world (Hawkins, "Charting Dante"). And so I am led to ask questions about my own book that only a few years ago I might not have thought to ask. What is its use? Whom can it benefit and how? What impact, if any, can such a study have on the rapidly changing patterns of medical practice today and—even more important—tomorrow?

For scholars, particularly literary theorists, students of popular culture, and sociologists, this book calls attention to a body of writings that should be of great interest. Literary critics will want to include pathography as a subgenre of autobiography and examine how it verifies or challenges various tenets of autobiographical theory. For example, pathography seems to challenge poststructuralist literary theories about the fictive reality of the self, to reinforce the current emphasis on the link between individual and culture, and to call into question the primacy so commonly attributed to gender.[1] For the cultural critic, a number of issues in my analysis of pathography call for further exploration: for example, the connection of the military myth to the pervasive violence of American society or the continuity between the mythos of healthy-mindedness and the current fad of self-help books and recovery programs. For the sociologist of medicine, pathography is a rich source for research into the changing relations of doctors and patients, the dramatic shift from positive to negative attitudes toward orthodox medicine and the evolving interest in alternative therapies, and the complex interplay of social expectations and medical practices as these impinge on the experiences and the imaginations of individual patients.

For teachers and administrators in our medical schools, my book and the pathographies it analyzes suggest the need for medical students to be better educated in the humanistic dimensions of medicine. What may be required is a drastic revision of medical education so that the ethical aspects of a medical situation are fully integrated into patient care, the individuality of the patient is recognized and honored both in theory and in practice, and the beliefs, assumptions, and attitudes of patients become an intrinsic concern in actual medical practice. I realize that such a call for reform is nothing new. The concern that contemporary Western medicine, in its emphasis on biochemistry and technology, is neglecting personal and social dimensions of illness has been voiced over and over for many years. A landmark of sorts in this call for reform is George Engel's essay in *Science* (1977), suggesting that a "biopsychosocial" model replace the traditional biomedical model. It is possible, though, that the implementation of such reforms may be more feasible now than ever before. In discussing very sick patients, physicians talk of "windows" within which they can intervene and possibly alter the course of the illness. Given the enormous changes facing medicine today—economic, political, social, ethical—there is a "window" of opportunity for medicine to reconstitute itself as a profession devoted primarily to the welfare of sick persons, rather than to the treatment of disease, as is the case now. The contribution pathography offers to such a project is obvious. I have found these books invaluable in teaching medical students, less perhaps to understand the experience of illness—for no written account can replicate what it is like to be ill—than to grasp the importance of the assumptions, attitudes, and myths that patients bring to the medical encounter. It is this encounter and the kind of interaction that issues from it that must be central to the science and art of medicine.

For people who are ill or concerned for a sick family member or friend, this book might serve as a "metapathography." Pathography provides a kind of vicarious support group, offering some guidance in the bewildering and often frightening terrain of serious illness. My account of particular pathographies might alert such people to books they would find personally helpful; at the same time, my analysis of myths about illness might encourage the use of those myths that can be enabling, while warning of the potential of any myth to prove disabling in a particular case. For those who care for the sick, an awareness of myths about illness is crucial: physicians clearly need to be able to identify myths such as these, even in latent or unconscious forms, to be sensitive to their depth and potential power, and to be aware of the capacity of such myths to help or to harm.

But it is in restoring the patient's voice to the medical enterprise that the study of pathography has its greatest importance and offers its greatest promise. For, as everyone realizes, we face a major crisis in medical practice at this moment. And this crisis, whose economic, political, and social dimensions are becoming as familiar as they are challenging, has a less recognized human dimension. It is surely no accident that the appearance of pathography coincides with the triumph of scientific technological medicine. The price we are paying for its remarkable achievements is felt by the individuals whose bodies can be so miraculously repaired, and it is a human price. We recognize this cost when patients fear their treatment more than their disease, when a hospital experience is compared to incarceration in a concentration camp, when the elderly are subjected—sometimes by family and sometimes by physicians—to processes that can only prolong dying at the price of indignity and suffering. Pathographies make such problems vividly and immediately real for us, and thus they have a significant part to play in the movement towards a patient-centered medicine.

ACKNOWLEDGMENTS

✤

I am indebted to the American Council of Learned Societies for awarding me a research fellowship in 1981–82, which helped me in the beginning stages of this project, and to the National Endowment for the Humanities for a fellowship (grant number FB-28585) supporting the completion of this book during the spring and summer of 1991. Howard Spiro provided me with an academic "home" as a visiting fellow at Yale University School of Medicine during the writing of portions of the manuscript, as did Wesleyan University's Graduate Liberal Studies Program and Center for the Humanities. I am especially grateful to David Barnard, chairman of the Department of Humanities at the Pennsylvania State University College of Medicine, who was willing to delay my appointment there so that I could accept the NEH grant and complete the book. A fine chairman and a good friend, he has supported me in this project in many ways.

I owe special debts of gratitude to Rita Charon and Debra Chwast, whose advice proved definitive in my decision to write the book at all; to Kathryn Montgomery Hunter, Joanne Trautmann Banks, and David Barnard, who read the entire manuscript in its final form and provided me with indispensable advice; to David J. Hufford, for his helpful comments on my last chapter; and to George R. Simms, who advised me as to medical idiom and practice. The flaws and errors that remain in the book are my own. I am grateful to Oliver Sacks for the encouragement he gave me in an interview during the very early stages of this project and for the constant inspiration provided me through my many readings of *Awakenings*. Endorsement of this project by Anne Hudson Jones, Rita Charon, and Philip Hallie helped me win NEH support. I am indebted to Barbara MacEachern and her staff at the Graduate Liberal Studies Program at Wesleyan University for their many kindnesses and to the Interlibrary Loan staff at Olin Library, Wesleyan University; the Hershey Public Library; and the George T. Harrell Library, Penn State College of Medicine, for their generous assistance. I am fortunate in my editor, Margaret Hunt.

With her enthusiasm, sense of humor, and background as a scholar, she has made the long process of turning a manuscript into a book almost a pleasure. Most of all I want to thank my husband, Sherman Hawkins, whose encouragement, patience, and love have sustained me through the years it took to complete this project and whose extraordinary insight has enabled me, like Diomedes in that other *aristeia,* to discern the gods from the mortals.

Lastly, I want to express my gratitude to all the authors whose pathographies I comment on in this book. I realize that I have taken what for them is a very personal story and analyzed it, sometimes critically. I ask their forgiveness if I have misinterpreted any portion of their work or distorted their meaning. I also ask them to understand that my aim in writing this book, like the stated aim of so many of these authors in their pathographies, is to help us all understand better what it means to have a chronic or life-threatening illness in America today.

Portions of the book have been published previously. The material on John Donne's *Devotions* in chapter 2 appeared in "Two Pathographies: A Study in Illness and Literature," *The Journal of Medicine and Philosophy* 9, no. 3 (August 1984), 231–52. © 1984 by Kluwer Academic Publishers.

A version of my discussion of the myth of rebirth and pathographies describing heart disease in chapter 2 appeared in "A Change in Heart: The Paradigm of Regeneration in Medical and Religious Narrative," *Perspectives in Biology and Medicine* 33, no. 4 (Summer 1990), 547–59. © 1990 by the University of Chicago.

Sections of chapter 4 appeared in "Constructing Death: Three Pathographies about Dying," *Omega* 22, no. 4 (1991), 301–17. © 1991 by Baywood Publishing Co., Inc.

My commentary on Gilda Radner's pathography in chapter 5 appeared in "Restoring the Patient's Voice: The Case of Gilda Radner," *The Yale Journal of Biology and Medicine* 65, no. 4 (1992). © The Yale Journal of Biology and Medicine, Inc.

The Society for Health and Human Values has provided a forum for my work more than once in addresses and speeches.

✦

CHAPTER ONE

Introduction

"*Robinson Crusoe*—that is what I think of. Surviving a terrible storm at sea; then being shipwrecked; waking from catastrophe and finding oneself alone in a new, alien, and dangerous world" (Pond, 4–5). This was written not by the survivor of a shipwreck but by a woman who suffered a brain tumor and the operation that removed it. Her book, entitled *Surviving,* is an example of what I call *pathography,*[1] a form of auto-biography or biography that describes personal experiences of illness, treatment, and sometimes death. "What it is like to have cancer" or "how I survived my heart attack" or "what it means to have AIDS"—these are the typical subjects of pathography. Such books are remarkably popular today: Gilda Radner's pathography about her cancer experience stayed on the *New York Times Book Review* best-seller list for months; Martha Weinman Lear's description of her physician-husband's long illness and eventual death from heart disease was available at supermarket checkout lanes; Norman Cousins's *Anatomy of an Illness,* an account of his recovery from a rare collagen disease using unorthodox therapeutic measures, is a book often found on a hospital patient's bedside table. And these are only a few examples of the many pathographies now in print.

In some sense, the pathography is our modern adventure story. Life becomes filled with risk and danger as the ill person is transported out of the familiar everyday world into the realm of a body that no longer functions and an institution as bizarre as only a hospital can be; life in all its myriad dimensions is reduced to a series of battles against death; and there is the inescapable sense, both for the sick person and his or her family, of being suddenly plunged into "essential" experience—the deeper realities of life. Given this presence of the dramatic and the terrifying, it is not so surprising that these "adventurers" are moved to write about their experiences. As Anatole Broyard observes, "Like anyone who has had an extraordinary experience, I wanted to describe it. . . . My initial experience of illness was as a series of disconnected shocks, and my first instinct was to try to bring it under control by turning it into a narrative" (21,19).

In their concern with illness, pathographies are like survival stories about natural or environmental disasters: the battle simply to stay alive despite exposure to shark-infested waters, or freezing temperatures, or marauding cancer cells, or antibodies that turn against the body that has produced them—these are all variations on a long-standing heroic paradigm of the struggle of brave individuals confronting what appear to be insurmountable forces. Since they also concern therapy, which is a cultural and not a natural activity, and hospitals, which are not jungles or oceans but societal institutions, pathographies can resemble accounts of political or racial oppression: one author remarks that her mother, hospitalized for cancer treatment, reminds her "of hostages and concentration camp prisoners who at first resist their captors and then try to appease them by good behavior" (Schreiber, 262).

Pathography offers us cautionary parables of what it would be like if our ordinary life-in-the-world suddenly collapsed. And indeed most of us, at some time or another, have recognized that the apparent orderliness and coherence of our lives is something of an accident, or a gift, or a miracle that renews itself day after day. Yet most of us behave as though this miracle were quite natural—a constant around which we can organize our lives. Thus we plan for the next day, and we go to sleep at night in confidence that the world (and we ourselves) will be the same the following morning. Pathographical narratives offer us a disquieting glimpse of what it is like to live in the absence of order and coherence. They show us the drastic interruption of a life of meaning and purpose by an illness that often seems arbitrary, cruel, and senseless; and by treatment procedures that too often can appear as likewise arbitrary, cruel, and senseless—especially to the person undergoing them. As one author of a pathography observes, "I exist in the world as most people see it, but I live in the world of the person with terminal cancer" (Shapiro, 130). Pathographies concern the attempts of individuals to orient themselves in the world of sickness—the world Susan Sontag calls "the kingdom of the sick" (1979, 3)—to achieve a new balance between self and reality, to arrive at an objective relationship both to experience and to the experiencing self. The task of the author of a pathography is not only to describe this disordering process but also to restore to reality its lost coherence and to discover, or create, a meaning that can bind it together again.

This need to bind things together again makes pathographical literature a rich source for the literary critic. My purpose here is to analyze pathography as illustrative of cultural myths, attitudes, and assumptions about various aspects of the illness experience in America today—the disease itself, therapy, recovery or death, medical personnel, and medical institutions.[2] In exploring these myths, I have for the most part limited my study to narratives that describe bodily (not psychiatric) illness, narratives that concern sickness (not disability or handicaps), and narratives that are written by or about an adult (not about children).[3] Another category of ill persons not represented in my book is the economically and socially disadvantaged—the poor and the homeless—a group that, to date, is minimally represented in pathographical literature. Each of the groups excluded could itself provide a subject worthy of a book-length study.

I will be treating pathography as a subgenre of autobiography, especially in the way I use literary theory, and will include as autobiography collaborative works as well as pathographies utilizing a journal format. Though some pathographies are technically biographies—narrative accounts of the death of a loved one—they are as much autobiographical accounts of the author's experience as witness as they are biographical accounts of another's illness and death. Unlike the case history or the conventional biography, with their supposedly disinterested perspective, biographical pathographies are almost always written by someone with a close relation to the ill person who is the book's subject, and thus they override the conventional boundaries of self and other or biographer and subject. Pathographies about an illness that has culminated in death form a part of the process of grieving: into the narrative of illness and death is interwoven the witnessing author's feelings, thoughts, and organizing images and metaphors, as he or she goes about the work of mourning.

An Overview of Pathography

As a genre, pathography is remarkable in that it seems to have emerged *ex nihilo;* book-length personal accounts of illness are uncommon before 1950 and rarely found before 1900. To do justice to the range and variety of these books is difficult. One way to organize them is in terms of disease categories—indeed, this is the way preferred by the Library of Congress.

Such an approach is useful in showing us which particular diseases are popular subjects for pathography. An informal EPIC computer search for titles from 1988 to 1992 reveals three entries under stroke, nine under heart disease, thirteen for multiple sclerosis, thirty-one for AIDS, and one hundred two for cancer (twenty-four of which refer to breast cancer). My concern here, however, is not with nomothetic generalizations about disease entities but with the way an individual deals with his or her illness—the myths, attitudes, and beliefs of our culture that a sick person uses to come to terms with illness. Though there are certain patterns specific to individual diseases—patterns that are discussed in the following chapters—it seems more appropriate that an overview of pathography should emphasize persons rather than their illnesses. Therefore, I will try to suggest some sense of the genre as a whole by flagging the author's explicit or implicit intent in writing the pathography.

If we use authorial intent as an organizing principle, pathographies tend to fall into three groups: testimonial pathographies, angry pathographies, and pathographies advocating alternative modes of treatment. Those in the first category, written for the most part in the late 1960s and the 1970s, are like religious "testimonies," public professions of faith that are meant to bear witness to the truth and strengthen other believers by relating an experience of spiritual trial or conversion. The intent of these pathographical testimonies seems to be simply to tell the story of an illness experience, focusing primarily on the author's thoughts, feelings, and behaviors as complementary to medical treatment that is generally accepted as appropriate and helpful. These books almost always project a positive attitude toward medicine. Since they are often written with the expressed purpose of helping others, pathographies in this first group can be seen as motivated by didactic or altruistic principles.

Pathographies written with an overtly didactic intent blend a personal account of illness with practical information. Descriptions of experience with breast cancer almost always fall into this category: these are books that have enabled women to be aware of therapeutic alternatives and to deal with postoperative trauma. An example is Marilyn Snyder's *An Informed Decision,* a book explicitly written for women with breast cancer who might be helped by surgical reconstruction. Joyce Slayton Mitchell's *Winning the Chemo Battle* is addressed to people undergoing chemotherapy, its stated goal being to help readers "plan and work toward your own quality of life" (10). Yet this same pathography also emphasizes the distinctiveness of its personal narrative: "If you have had chemotherapy, you will recognize the 'truth' in this book, even though your own may be different" (9). Other didactic pathographies are concerned with negotiating changes in life-style. Thus Bea Keiser's *All Our Hearts Are Trump* concerns the adjustments her family has had to make when her husband suffers a heart attack. The book is a kind of manual for families of heart-attack victims, giving advice on everything from reassessing values to changes in eating habits. Another example of didactic pathography is Herbert Conley's *Living and Dying Gracefully*. The book, "written for all those who are presently walking a similar path" (x), is just what its title suggests, a sort of manual that blends the author's own experience in confronting pain and death with what he has learned in his role as minister to sick and dying parishioners.

Pathographies of this kind are often written with the expectation that the author's experience might serve as a mirror, or a model, for the prospective reader. Thus authors with heart disease will direct their narratives to potential readers with heart disease; women writing about breast cancer will write for other women with the same problem. To some extent this assumption of the "generalizability" of illness is a part of our modern nomothetic mythology about disease, which assumes a uniformity of experience within a diagnostic category.

At the end of the 1970s, pathographies begin to change dramatically in tone and intent. Trust in physicians and tolerance of hospital routines are no longer the norm but now the exception; in fact, they are replaced by a striking lack of confidence in physicians and an overt fear of hospitalization. Pathographies written in the 1980s signal an important cultural shift away from several of midcentury America's favorite cultural myths: that of the medical encounter as comforting and reassuring—a myth perfectly epitomized in the popular Norman Rockwell image of a portly, benign, and paternal physician ministering to a snub-nosed child—and that of medical science as invincible in its march to eradicate disease, a myth celebrated in the *Reader's Digest*'s "Miracles of Modern Medicine."

Recent pathographies demonstrate our cultural discontent with traditional medicine in two different ways: by the expression of anger at callous or needlessly depersonalizing medical treatment and by a concern with alternative medical therapies. Both suggest a revolt against the benign medical mythology communicated on the covers of the *Saturday Evening Post* or in the pages of the *Reader's Digest*. Moreover, both reflect and help create a new cultural attitude, one which recognizes that the onset of serious illness brings with it not only problems occasioned by the illness itself but also problems caused by therapies, by the medical institution where treatment takes place, and by the physicians who oversee that treatment. As one author observes during a lengthy hospitalization, "I was no longer afraid of the disease, but of the system" (Baier, 100).

Angry pathographies are intended to expose and denounce atrocities in the way illness is treated in America today. These books testify to a medical system seen as out of control, dehumanized, and sometimes brutalizing; and they are written from a sense of outrage over particular and concrete instances of what is perceived to be the failure of medicine to care adequately for the ill. So one author, in a section that begins, "I hate Mom's doctors," expresses with great bitterness her frustration at the way her mother's physicians fail to deal with pain. Doctors, she observes, "are specialists trained to intervene at moments of crisis, to cut, to radiate, to alter chemistry, then move on to the next patient. But why is there no place in this elaborate medical system for sustained care of the human being who continues to feel the effects of the doctors' knives and beams and chemicals?" (Schreiber, 138). Another author, hospitalized for cancer treatment, observes: "I find myself apologizing for being a person rather than a case, for having feelings and wanting—needing—to understand what they are doing to me . . . what is happening to me" (Cook, 209). Yet another author writes: "The first urologist . . . I saw treated me as if I were a specimen. Instead of speaking to me after he examined my testicle, he called over a resident, pointed out a 'calcification' . . . and began talking to him about 'surgery'" (Fiore, 3).

In a sense, these are "case histories" of the way Western scientific medicine is practiced today, especially in the United States. Two factors emerge again and again in these "cases": the tendency in contemporary medical practice to focus primarily not on the needs of the individual who is sick but on the nomothetic condition that we call disease, and the sense that our medical technology has advanced beyond our capacity to use it wisely. These books show how an ill person today can be both the beneficiary and the victim of a health-care system whose very excellence—its superb technological achievements—is at the same time potentially dehumanizing.

The angry pathographies seem to begin in 1980 with Martha Weinman Lear's very popular *Heartsounds*, a book that painfully and bitterly catalogues everything that went wrong during her physician-husband's many hospitalizations for heart disease and every way in which his doctors failed him. The book begins with irony, as she describes *Doctor* Lear's confident diagnosis of a pain in his chest as heartburn and not heart attack (it is a misdiagnosis). The author goes on to describe an infection that results from an intern's refusal to attend to a minor inflammation from a needle, a coronary angiography where anesthesia is given after the procedure is completed, and another occasion when severe irritation of the stomach lining results from huge doses of potassium given without liquids; it describes a doctor who gives wrong medical advice and then blames the patient for his own mistakes, and other doctors who wish their patient dead when they have done all that they can and he does not recover. The book ends as it began with a medical failure—the failure of the autopsy report to provide the "answers," the medical explanations that Ms. Lear so desperately feels she needs. Overall, the book leaves us with the sense of a man and his wife victimized by a medical system consistently portrayed as incompetent and uncaring.

A more recent pathography of this kind is Sue Baier's *Bed Number Ten*, an angry description of callous and indifferent treatment by medical personnel during her long stay in an intensive care unit. The book is prefaced by a brief but bitter statement, allotted an entire page: "The names of the hospital and all medical personnel have been changed to protect those who were less than kind." Her anger is directed not at the medical management of the course of her disease, which seems to have been exemplary, but at the impersonal, dehumanizing way in which she is treated. Afflicted with Guillain-Barré syndrome, Baier is totally paralyzed but also totally conscious. Thus she is in a terribly vulnerable position: she retains normal sensitivity to pain, but since she cannot move or talk, lacks any way to signal when she feels it. The actual incidents of mistreatment she records seem relatively minor, taken separately. They include such unnecessarily painful nursing procedures as flushing out her ears with cold water and cleaning her mouth with undiluted peroxide, and the way her physicians repeatedly ignore the fact that she is conscious and sentient. These minor mistreatments, she believes, together add up to a style of medical care that seems to disregard the reality of bodily pain and consistently ignores the subjective dimension of illness. Baier asks, "Was I paranoid to want to be treated as human? To be asked how I felt? Did you sleep well, Sue? Are you comfortable? . . . There were so many little things, constantly, one after the other—indignities that led to my desperation" (194).

Another kind of experience that can result in an angry pathography begins with the cancer patient's search for the "top" cancer specialist and the "best" research protocol. One such book is Jean Craig's *Hello and Goodbye,* the story of her fifty-nine-year-old husband's decision to "fire" the oncologist who offers him little hope for reversing a cancer of the colon metastasized to both lungs, and his subsequent determination to hunt down promising cancer treatments. After several interviews and examinations, Craig decides on a particular protocol and enrolls in a randomized cancer trial with a very new, very experimental regimen. All goes well, despite the terrible side effects of his treatment, until it becomes evident that his illness is not going to be reversed. At this point the Craigs respond with bitterness and increasing anger toward his doctors for their reluctance to share pertinent information, their sense of "entitlement," their indifference to their patient's comfort, their emotional remoteness, their focus on the disease and not the patient, and their "insultingly, offensively patronizing" answers to questions posed by patient and family (305). The anger in this pathography stems from the Craigs' sense of betrayal in their conviction—a conviction encouraged and possibly shared by the research oncologists whom they seek out—that an aggressive, militant approach to cancer will result in a cure. As one research oncologist whom they consult points out, the difference between medical research and medical practice is the difference between doctors who "attack" and doctors who "treat" (21). In a sense, the Craigs get what they thought they wanted.

Pathographies like these, however, while not infrequent, are really not characteristic of the genre, though they do seem to be the pathographies highlighted in the media. In fact, not many pathographies are dominated by a need to expose the outrages of modern medicine—"doctor-bashing," as this is sometimes described. Most pathographies do include criticisms of doctors or therapies or hospital care, but they include praise as well. It is important to remember that the focus in most pathography is really not on the medical enterprise, whether this is judged to be good or bad, but on patient experience. And patient experience includes a good many dimensions beyond conventional medical treatment: the subjective aspects of illness; its effect on family, friends, and work; alternative therapies and the individuals associated with them; and exposure through the media to lay and pseudoscientific understandings of illness and treatment. Increasingly, the medical establishment is only one part of an illness experience.

The third group of pathographies begins with Norman Cousins's popular *Anatomy of an Illness,* published as a book in 1979 (and before that as an article in the *New England Journal of Medicine* in 1976). Like their angry counterparts, these pathographies seem to stem from a sense of dissatisfaction with the way medicine is practiced today. They differ, though, in that their authors are concerned not so much with criticizing traditional medicine as with finding alternative treatment modalities—modalities that sometimes supplement traditional therapies and sometimes replace them altogether. These books reveal a patient population empowered by a belief in the nearly limitless capacities of the mind and the emotions to facilitate healing, and eager to find some objective correlative in holistic therapies to the inner resources of psyche and spirit.

The authors of these pathographies assume that therapeutic success derives in part (some would say primarily) from the patient's attitude—the "will to live" that has by now become a battle cry for many ill people. Moreover many, like Cousins, assume that the will to live is actually based in physiology, a notion that challenges the Cartesian dualism of mind and body that has been a cornerstone of modern scientific medicine. Growing support for this position—that mind and body are interrelated and that healing always involves an interplay between mental and physical—can be found in the new science of psychoneuroimmunology and in the many forms of alternative medicine now available.

Unlike the angry pathographies, with their predilection for "doctor-bashing," pathographies concerned with alternative therapies commonly project a positive attitude toward the author's physicians. Even so, this positive attitude goes hand in hand with a sense of the diminished importance of the physician and of orthodox medicine in general. Indeed, orthodox medicine is accorded the role in the world of illness that medicine itself tends to claim as its rightful province—attention to biochemical aspects of bodily structure and function. And the biochemical is felt by these patients to be only one aspect of treating illness and maintaining health. Mental attitude, nutrition, exercise, response to stress, even personal and societal goals and values—these are judged at least as important as the narrow biochemical focus of orthodox medicine. Pathographies written in the 1980s fairly bristle with holistic and alternative therapies—therapies ranging from such relatively conventional practices as attention to diet and exercise, acupuncture, and visualization exercises to more unusual treatments: the use of quartz crystals, lucid dreams, and various naturopathic remedies.

Underlying the differing purposes of all three kinds of pathographies is a common motive—the need to communicate a painful, disorienting, and isolating experience. Indeed, the need to come to terms with a traumatic experience often involves the need to project it outwards—to talk or write about it. As Max Lerner observes of his own motive for writing a pathography: "I passed through a searing experience that tested and changed me in ways I never foresaw. And like the Ancient Mariner I want to tell my story, to whatever listeners it finds" (20). Though few patients do go on to write book-length narratives about their experience, the urge to tell others seems to be a common response to medical trauma. The intensity with which a casual acquaintance will describe his or her illness, especially when it involves hospitalization, is familiar to all of us. Pathography, then, can be seen as a literary expression of this need.

Furthermore, if there is a strong need to tell about one's own illness, there would also appear to be a strong urge to read about the illness of others. The proof of this is the remarkable popularity of pathographies. For the thousands who read them, pathographies serve as models suggesting attitude and behavior during illness. Lucy Shapero's *Never Say Die* provides a convincing example: it is a book directly inspired by another book, Cousins's *Anatomy of an Illness*. Other authors, too, will at times mention the impact of a pathography they have read. Le Anne Schreiber quotes Sontag's metaphor of illness as a "more onerous citizenship" (in *Illness as Metaphor*), using it to discuss the way she feels set apart by her immersion in her mother's sickness (70). David A. Tate in his pathography describes the way he uses Cousins's *The Healing Heart* in preparing for a postcoronary treadmill test; Lenor Madruga cites Betty Rollin's pathography about breast cancer; Beata Bishop is encouraged by Jaquie Davison's *Cancer Winner: How I Purged Myself of Melanoma* to begin her own detoxification diet.

Not all pathographies so used may be helpful, however. The pathography cited in *Heartsounds* is ominously appropriate to what happens to Harold Lear: after his heart attack and after heart surgery that results in brain damage, Lear reads a magazine article entitled "The Unnecessary Death of My Wife"—a story about a woman who undergoes open-heart surgery and dies from a series of postoperative mistakes (196). A different though also negative response to reading pathographies is discussed in Barbara Webster's *All of a Piece*. Webster, when she finds out she has multiple sclerosis, reads the pathographies about her disease but finds them unhelpful—limited by a too-narrow focus on the physical adjustments required, as well as unrealistically optimistic and hopeful in outlook.

For readers who are themselves ill, pathography articulates the hopes, fears, and anxieties so common to sickness, organizing them into a coherent whole and suggesting by example ways of thinking and acting. Didactic pathographies are read as guidebooks on how to find a good doctor or how to buy a prosthesis or how to adapt one's life-style to a heart attack; angry pathographies legitimize patients' demands for more humane medical care; pathographies describing alternative medical treatments alert ill persons to the fact that there are other ways of treating sickness and encourage their use. And for readers who are not themselves sick, pathography serves a preparatory function, so that when they do encounter some life-threatening illness (and most of us eventually will), this experience will inevitably be informed by what they have read.

In its capacity to serve as a model for others, pathography plays an important role in the way it both reflects and helps shape our current mythology about illness. As I hope to show, pathography embodies dynamic constructs about how to deal with disease and treatment: its images and metaphors and myths are not just decorative and fanciful but highly influential models of how to negotiate an illness experience.

Pathography as the Patient's Voice

It is striking that autobiographical descriptions of illness should belong almost exclusively to the second part of the twentieth century. Though in previous eras diaries and journals can be found in abundance, few of these take the author's experience of illness as their only subject. Why should this be so? One explanation is that in earlier times illness seems to have been considered an integral and inseparable part of living (and dying)—illness thus takes its place in journals and autobiographies along with other facets of a life. It is only in the twentieth century that serious illness has become a phenomenon that can be isolated from an individual's life—perhaps because such illness is set apart from normal life by hospitalization or perhaps because we now tend to consider health as the norm and illness as a condition to be corrected, never simply accepted.

Yet another way to look at the popularity of pathography today is to see it as a reaction to our contemporary medical model, one so dominated by a biophysical understanding of illness that its experiential aspects are virtually ignored. Medicine today has been criticized for its narrow focus on disease and its disregard for the experiencing patient. One result of so divorcing spirit or personality from body is that the experiential side of illness is relegated to the category of the epiphenomenal. The patient, observes Richard Baron, is in a sense "subtracted out" of the medical paradigm: "One obtains the idea of a pure disease which is, ideally, distinct from any particular patient. The disease manifests itself through the patient, and the patient comes to function as a kind of translucent screen on which the disease is projected" (7–8). Pathography restores the person ignored or canceled out in the medical enterprise, and it places that person at the very center. Moreover, it gives that ill person a voice.

Pathography, then, returns the voice of the patient to the world of medicine, a world where that voice is too rarely heard, and it does so in such a way as to assert the phenomenological, the subjective, and the experiential side of illness. What the voice of the patient tells us can be shocking, enlightening, or surprising. Is it possible that a highly respected hospital can be so deficient in patient care that needless suffering is caused by the indifference or incompetence of medical personnel? According to *Heartsounds*, this is what happened to Harold Lear. Is it possible to disregard conventional medical advice and recover from a severe illness by generous doses of laughter and vitamin C? In *Anatomy of an Illness*, Norman Cousins assures us that he did. Is it possible that a man with advanced, metastatic prostate cancer should enter remission by following a rigid macrobiotic diet? Physician-author Anthony Sattilaro in *Recalled by Life* reports that this is what happened to him.

In a sense, the pathography written by the patient or a loved one can be seen as the logical counterpart to the medical history written by the physician or by the medical staff assigned to a particular patient.[4] It would seem that they should be very similar, since both genres are concerned with the sickness and treatment of a specific individual. In fact, however, they are radically different in subject, purpose, structure, authorial persona, and tone.

The subject of the case report is a particular biomedical condition, the individual reduced to a body and the body reduced to its biophysical components ("the disease in the body in the bed"), while the true subject of pathography is illness and treatment as experienced and understood by the ill person who is its author. The purpose of the case report is to record diagnosis and treatment; the purpose of pathography is to draw out the meaning of the author's experience. The medical report is usually composed of brief factual statements about present symptoms and body chemistry, whereas a pathography is an extended narrative situating the illness experience within the author's life and the meaning of that life. The ideal medical report disavows any authorship at all (the first person pronoun is almost never used); on the other hand, the authorship of a pathography is never in question. Moreover the ideal case report omits any reference to the emotions either of physician or of patient. As Baron observes, the physician is encouraged to ignore the intuitive insight, the obvious observation, the common-sense solution—all in the service of an ideal of scientific objectivity. Pathography, at the other extreme, tends to focus on the emotional components of a medical experience, sometimes with unavoidably theatrical results.

Pathographies do tend to dramatize the events of illness. The drama in pathography, however, is no worse a distortion of reality than is the biomedical myopia of the case report. Indeed, if pathography is compared to the case report, the patient's own account will appear not so much a grossly exaggerated rendition of what happened as a corrective to the stark, depersonalized account of tests and procedures written up by medical personnel. Case report and pathography function as mirrors set at an oblique angle to experience: each one distorts, each one tells the truth.

An analysis of pathographical narrative suggests that a medical model which aims at rendering the patient transparent so that the physician may focus more clearly on the disease may indeed be misguided. Physicians sometimes need to be reminded that "disease" cannot exist apart from a diseased person: as Kathryn Montgomery Hunter observes, medicine is first and foremost "a science of individuals" (1989, 193). Pathography is a narrative reminder of this all-too-easily-neglected truth. The need somehow to put the patient back into the medical enterprise—to return the experiencing, suffering human being from the periphery to the center of medicine—this is the burden of many recent studies.

Elliot Mishler, writing about the medical interview, remarks on the way "the voice of the life-world" (the psychological and sociocultural contexts of a patient's experience) is dominated by "the voice of medicine" (a technological, bioscientific frame of reference). Rita Charon describes the way she implements Mishler's critique in an unusual method of teaching interviewing skills to medical students: she has them write semifictional accounts of an interview *using the patient's own voice,* in an attempt to restore to the medical encounter that "voice of the life-world." In *The Illness*

Narratives, Arthur Kleinman asserts that good clinical care involves not only the recognition of the patient's "explanatory model" of his or her illness but the affirmation of that model and the ability to incorporate it into an effective therapeutic approach. In this explanatory model, which is usually tacit, Kleinman includes all aspects of the patient's understanding of illness: what it is, why it happened, and what is expected or hoped for in regard to treatment.[5] Howard Brody, in *Stories of Sickness,* is similarly concerned with the need to restore patient experience to a position of primacy in the medical encounter, though he approaches the subject from the standpoint of a philosopher. Eric Cassell, in *The Nature of Suffering,* observes that "a shift is now taking place in medicine away from a primary concern with diseases and towards a focus on ill persons" (81). He urges that to complete this shift, "the concept of person" replace the Cartesian dualism basic to contemporary biomedicine. In all these books, there is a recognition of the need in medicine to perceive patients not in terms of laboratory tests and fever charts but in relation to their lives as persons. Pathography records the voice of the ill person: it is thus the exemplary illness narrative, the missing part of the patient history.

Autobiographical Theory and the "Truth" of Pathography

If it is true that pathography restores to the therapeutic paradigm the missing voice of the patient—the phenomenological, the experiential dimension of illness—then one may be tempted to assert that the patient narrative gives us the "true" or "real" story of what the experience was actually like. And we all share, to some extent, in the intuitive assumption that the person to whom the experience occurred is in the best position to describe it truthfully. Pathographies may indeed be read as "true stories," but the emphasis must be as much on the word "stories" as the word "true." For these books cannot be taken as accurate records of experience: they are too highly charged, as the ambivalence and prosaic quality of everyday living is resolved into sharp contrasts and clear-cut issues.

To emphasize the "story" element in these narratives is in no way to denigrate their truth-value. It is important, though, in analyzing pathography, to remember that the narrative description of illness is both less and more than the actual experience: less, in that remembering and writing are selective processes—certain facts are dropped because they are forgotten or because they do not fit the author's narrative design; and more, in that the act of committing experience to narrative form inevitably confers upon it a particular sequence of events and endows it with a significance that was probably only latent in the original experience. Narrative form alters experience, giving it a definite shape, organizing events into a beginning, a middle, and an end, and adding drama—heightening feelings and seeing the individuals involved as characters in a therapeutic plot. Writing about an experience—any experience—inevitably changes it.

The assertion that there is a significant difference between the original "real" experience and the retrospective autobiographical narrative is now a commonplace among critics and theorists of autobiography. Most critics see this difference as caused by the author's creative imposition of order, pattern, and meaning on what is remembered of one's life. Thus in *Design and Truth in Autobiography*, Roy Pascal discusses autobiography not as a chronicle but as an interpretation of a life. Pascal emphasizes that the way the autobiographer shapes the past reflects the author's particular standpoint at the moment of writing. The past, then, is not simply recorded in the autobiographical act but given a structure, a coherence, a meaning. Thus the process of autobiographical recollection is part self-discovery and part self-creation.

Pascal's careful qualifications about the factual authenticity of autobiography seem to have ignited a fierce critical skepticism about the ontological status of the autobiographical self and its past. The once solid self of autobiography now dissolves into a shimmer of critical qualifiers: we have Richard Olney's *Metaphors of Self*, Michael Sprinker's "Fictions of the Self," John Morris's *Versions of the Self*, Patricia Meyer Spacks's *Imagining a Self*, John O. Lyons's *The Invention of the Self*. In the last decade or so, the similarity between the task of psychoanalytic reconstruction and that of autobiographical reconstruction has come to seem almost an identity. Borrowing from recent psychoanalytic insights, autobiographical critics question our assumption "that a person's life is recoverable, all 'there' ready to be unearthed and transplanted" or maintain that "the past does not exist. There are memories of it—scattered shards of events and feelings—but they are re-created within a later context" (Mandel 1972, 324; Pike, 337).

An even more extreme viewpoint doubts not just the existence of the past but also the existence of the self, seeing it as a fiction of language. The self, claims Robert Elbaz, belongs to "the dimension of imagination and not of memory, an entity that must be renewed ceaselessly" (144). As James Cox observes about recent critical theory: "Language is thus the signifier presumptively making the self it signifies increasingly so absent that it can only be traced like a ghost between the long sequence of lines and text that make up a convention or a tradition" (3). So seen, the self is total invention—the only reality being the literary artifact: "the text takes on a life of its own, and the self that was not really in existence in the beginning is in the end merely a matter of text and has nothing whatever to do with an authorizing author" (Olney 1980, 22).

The question whether the self is a category prior to language or a construct of language is at present (and not surprisingly) still unresolved, but some critical approaches are able to move beyond this question without entirely dismissing it. One critical position that simply bypasses the issue of the fictional status of the self is the focus on what Elizabeth Bruss calls the "truth-value" of the autobiographical report and Philippe Lejeune, the "autobiographical pact." This pact is an explicit commitment of the author not to try to replicate all the facts of his or her life but to try instead to offer an understanding of that life: the "aim is not simple verisimilitude, but resemblance to the truth. Not 'the effect of the real,' but the image of the real" (Lejeune, 22).

Another critical viewpoint explains (and protects) the now fragile self by endowing it with a mystic ineffability. Thus Leo Braudy, writing about Defoe, refers to the autobiographical subject as "the mystery at the heart of human personality" (95); Germaine Brée, writing of Michel Leiris, alludes to the "inner self" of autobiography as a "center around which all else is articulated" though itself unreachable through language and as belonging "to the enigmatic realm of the 'sacred'" (200–201); and Barrett Mandel sees autobiographical reflection as the discovery of "the mysteriousness of [the author's] own existence" (1972, 323) and roots autobiography in "the deeper reality of being" (1980, 50).

Still other critics emphasize the difference between the author-self and the protagonist-self of autobiography. Louis Renza distinguishes between authorial person and authorial persona, alluding to the "split intentionality" in autobiographical writing whereby the "I" becomes a "he" (279). Paul John Eakin has it both ways: he prefaces *Fictions in Autobiography* with the assertion that "the self that is the center of all autobiographical narrative is necessarily a fictive structure," but elsewhere in the book he claims, "I regard the self finally as a mysterious reality, mysterious in its nature and origins and not necessarily consubstantial with the fictions we use to express it" (3, 277).

Most recently, the issue is again bypassed by implying an ideological and political, if not an ontological primacy for social and cultural reality over the much-disputed reality of selfhood. In a sense this marks a return to Roy Pascal, who remarked, more than thirty years ago, that autobiography "involves the philosophical assumption that the self comes into being only through interplay with the outer world" (8). So Albert Stone, arguing against the recent tendency to treat autobiography solely as a fictive enterprise, cites as equally important the "complex processes of historical re-creation, ideological argument, and psychological expression" (19). Considered as "social document," autobiography, he observes, "affords a special kind of information about a culture and the individuals embedded in it" (7, 6). In similar fashion, Burton Pike observes that certain contemporary autobiographers "take their present experiences and attitudes as representative of certain forces at work in their culture"—a stance that he calls "extrospective" (342).[6]

Thus in autobiographical criticism and theory, three central issues emerge: the question of the ontological status of the self; the "extrospective" social and cultural dimensions; and the question of whether the past is reflected, reordered, or created in the act of writing about it. Pathography offers its own perspective on these various critical stances. First, in regard to the autobiographical self: neither the self as fiction nor the self as ineffable mystery are adequate formulations for the self encountered in pathographical narrative. In narratives describing illness and death, the reader is repeatedly confronted with the pragmatic reality and experiential unity of the autobiographical self. Pathography challenges the skepticism of critics and theorists about the self, making that skepticism seem artificial, mandarin, and contrived. The self of pathographical writing is the self-in-crisis: when confronted with serious and life-threatening illness, those possibilities, fictions, metaphors, and versions of self are contracted into a "hard" defensive ontological reality—primed for action, readied for response to the threat of the body, alternatively resisting and inviting the eventual disintegration of the self that is death. Perhaps it is true, as Freud maintained, that the ego is first and foremost a bodily ego and that "self" is bound up with the biological integrity of the body.

Second, pathography validates a critical stance that emphasizes the importance of sociocultural elements in writings about the self. Pierre Macherey and others see a text not as a creation by an author but as a product of a society, with the authorial role diminished to that of a facilitator, or producer. Pathographies support this emphasis on society and culture, though they do so in a way that does not diminish or efface the self. For illness in pathography is always experienced in relation to a particular con-figuration of cultural ideologies, practices, and attitudes—and these inform the various components of our health-care system: professional personnel, particular diagnostic tests and particular therapies, and institutions such as the hospital and the clinic. All pathographies, even those that eventually discard traditional medical approaches, are situated within the social praxis of modern medicine; therefore, they all can serve as commentaries on it.

Lastly, if pathography challenges recent critical skepticism about the self and confirms the recent emphasis on cultural context, it significantly ad-vances the critical position about autobiography as a re-creation of the past. As most autobiographical theorists maintain, the past in any autobiogra-phy is not simply recorded but is changed, reordered, even re-created in the act of writing about it. The study of pathography is important to this po-sition because it discloses the particular ways in which the author changes the experiences he or she claims to be faithfully documenting. As I will show, this change is one that, in achieving a formulation of the experience that the author finds satisfying, exposes certain metaphoric and mythic constructs about illness in our culture.

Mythic Thinking

As we have seen, the "pathographical act" is one that constructs meaning by subjecting raw experience to the powerful impulse to make sense of it all, to bind together the events, feelings, thoughts, and sensations that oc-cur during an illness into an integrated whole. Pathographies answer the need for what Sam Banks has called "meaningful, satisfying closures in a slippery world always threatening to open at the seams" (24). It is this con-structive aspect of the autobiographical act—autobiography in its creative dimensions—that is the object of my concern in this book. Pathographies interpret experience, and they do so in a way that discloses certain impor-tant mythic attitudes about illness and treatment. Mythic thinking of all kinds becomes apparent in that delicate autobiographical transition from "actual" experience to written narrative, since this transition is one that constructs necessary fictions out of the building blocks of metaphor, im-age, archetype, and myth. Furthermore, as I hope to show, these heuristic mythologies of illness are formative: they serve not only to organize expe-rience and to open it up to interpretation but also to shape it.

This word *myth* is problematic but necessary to my analysis of path-ography and, thus, requires further explanation. Today, *myth* has two contradictory meanings: the first (and probably more common) definition is *illusion* or *fiction,* the second refers to a deeper significance or a more profound truth. Myths are illusory or fictive in that they are epiphenomenal: the myth of progress, for example, is a conceptual scheme superimposed on human history, but it does not describe human history itself. On the other hand, myths are profound in that they embody significant patterns of human thought and behavior that emerge in cultural practices and beliefs: the myth of renewal, for example, is reflected in rituals of initiation both ancient and modern. I use the word *myth* in discussing pathography in both these senses of illusion and profound truth.[7]

Plato's use of myth in his dialogues is an ancient but still valid example of the mythic as inclusive of contradictory meanings. The *Euthyphro* is a dialogue between Socrates and Euthyphro, a young priest who is about to demonstrate what he considers his outstanding piety by bringing suit against his own father. As proof of the exemplary nature of this action, Euthyphro first refers to Zeus, "the best and most just of the gods," who punished his father, Kronos, with imprisonment, and then to Kronos before him, who punished his father with castration. Socrates responds that he finds it hard to believe such stories and observes that this is why he, Socrates, is being prosecuted for impiety by the state. The point that Plato is making is that myths like these are fantastic, fictive, and certainly not true in any literal sense. Yet in a deeper-than-literal sense, the dialogue demonstrates that the myth *is* true: Euthyphro is the living embodiment of this myth—he is acting out the myth of the son who turns on his own father. And though Euthyphro appears a fool for his naive belief in stories like this, he is a dangerous fool, for he is a type of the pious citizen who will execute Socrates for not believing the stories about the gods as literally true. For Plato, then, a myth is at one level a fictional story about the gods and, at a deeper level, a figural narrative that points toward a universal truth or pattern of behavior. At this deeper level, myth is not explanation but embodiment, a "symbolic activity where the symbol participates in what it represents" (Dardel, 45). Moreover at this level, the mythic is conceived as functional, as dynamic.

In modern times, though, myth is often seen as something that is invented or imagined. This notion of myth as invention was one encouraged by the "science" of mythology, originating in the nineteenth century and represented by such scholars as the anthropologist Edward Tylor. Writing out of a Darwinian perspective, Tylor conceives of myth as stories invented by the "savage" to explain the world around him. Mythology here is understood as primitive science or false science; the myth of Apollo the sun-god driving his chariot through the heavens each day is thus an explanation of the perceived motion of the sun, a story that is at the same time fictional, mythic, and pseudoscientific. Our contemporary notion of myth as a fiction derives from this nineteenth-century academic understanding of mythology as a false, incorrect explanation of how the world works—an explanation now replaced by science, which supposedly offers the only true and correct account.

For many scholars and thinkers today, from a great many varied disciplines, myth is not an explanatory fiction but a way of articulating deep personal and cultural truths. Freud and Jung are seminal figures in this restoration of myth to the status of embodied truth: the Oedipal myth is central to Freud's theory of sexuality; quest myths are key to Jung's emphasis on spiritual fulfillment in realizing the true self. Though a full discussion of modern theories of myth is beyond the purview of this book, it may be helpful to suggest the variety of thinkers who use myth in this way. There are myth critics Mircea Eliade and Joseph Campbell; anthropologists Claude Lévi-Strauss, Arnold van Gennep, and Victor Turner; philosophers Ernst Cassirer, Lucien Lévy-Bruhl, and Leszek Kolakowski; theologian Rudolf Bultmann; and literary critics Northrop Frye, Maud Bodkin, Philip Wheelwright, and Roland Barthes.[8]

For Cassirer, the mythic is a primary and irreducible element in human thinking. Myth is expressive, not explanatory: as he observes, "The 'image' does not represent the 'thing'; it *is* the thing; it does not merely stand for the object, but has the same actuality" (38). For Bultmann, myth must be interpreted anthropologically, or existentially: "the real point of myth is not to give an objective world picture; what is expressed in it, rather, is how we human beings understand ourselves in our world" (9).[9] For Wheelwright, the mythic is a way of thinking, a way of knowing, a way of perceiving: it is not "a fiction imposed on one's already given world, but . . . a way of apprehending that world"—a "radically cognitive" act. The mythic offers a unique perspective on things, "a set of depth-meanings of perduring significance" that transcend the limits of what can be expressed in ordinary speech (159).

What all these thinkers share is the understanding of myth as embodied truth. I suggest that myth and its function be further defined as integrative, as connective, and as analogical. First, myth is integrative in that it involves a synthesizing activity of mind: it does not break up experience into its component parts but brings it together into unity, organizing experience into a unified whole. Second, myth relates the particular and individual to some larger dimension. Though myths are usually transcultural and transhistorical, they can also be related to a particular culture or subculture. Whatever the circumference of the particular mythos, it always places events and characters in a wider context, so that the individual is part of the whole and the particular is seen in relation to the universal. Third, myth substitutes analogy for explicit meaning. Meaning in the usual sense seems almost irrelevant to myth, since the meaning of a myth is not something articulated but something felt or apprehended: in the dimension of the mythic, meaning is encoded in metaphor. A myth thus does not interpret or explain; it works analogically to embody or picture meaning. Not surprisingly, its primary epistemic devices are the image, symbol, and archetype. It is these elements, then, that will be central to my analysis of mythic thinking in pathography.

The myths about illness that one finds in pathographies may well be fictions, in the sense that when people write about their "journey" into the realm of illness, they may have traveled no further than their local hospital. But myths about illness must also be seen as profound truth in that they describe the inner configuration of the ill person's experience. For example, the myth of illness as a battle between two opposed forces is the way illness *is* actually experienced by a surprisingly large number of people who write pathographies and by some of the even larger number of people who read them.

In addition to seeing myths about illness as both fictive and profoundly true, it is important that we recognize the *dynamic* nature of myth—its potential impact on every dimension of an illness experience. Cassirer stresses this dynamic aspect of the mythic, observing: "It is not by its history that the mythology of a nation is determined but, conversely, its history is determined by its mythology . . ." (5). Myths about illness not only reflect experience but they also determine its actual shape. For example, if individuals perceive their illness as an adversary, an enemy to be defeated, then they usually acquiesce to any and all therapies their doctors deem possible "weapons." This is a myth that is medically syntonic; that is, consistent with the metaphors and myths inherent in Western medicine. However, if the ill person believes that the key to recovery from illness is right attitude, then the effectiveness of purely medical treatments is more questionable. This is a myth that, for obvious reasons, can be at times medically dystonic.

Myths about illness are not restricted to the patient population: physicians also have their myths about illness, though these may not be the same as those held by their patients. And doctor myths are just as powerful as patient myths, or perhaps more so. For example, the metaphor of the human body as a machine, a metaphor basic to contemporary biomedicine, is itself a kind of mythic thinking. In pathography, the mechanistic myth quite often works dystonically to create an impasse between what the patient actually feels and what can be determined by chemical analyses and technological monitors. Too often, symptoms for which physicians can find no organic cause (and which are thus often considered untreatable) are in one way or another simply dismissed. So one pathographer writes about a subjective condition experienced as "fog": "The thing fits no clinical profile. It yields no diagnosis. It submits to none of their tests, invites no techniques, and so what are they to do?. . . Whatever cannot be diagnosed or treated by technique is suspect, vaguely inauthentic, and quite possibly does not exist" (Lear, 187). The mechanistic metaphor so central to Western medicine has little place for the subjective components of body function. How patients feel, their understanding of what is happening to them, and the sense of how their illness may alter their lives are peripheral to a mechanistic model.[10]

Although contemporary medical theory and practice are rife with analogical thinking of all kinds, the ideal of modern medicine is to eschew mythic thinking at every level. Thus it is recognized that the less a phenomenon is fully (i.e., scientifically) understood, the more it tends to be described in metaphoric language; correspondingly, the more it is understood, the fewer concessions need to be made to image and metaphor. The medical ideal, then, is a language fully purged of mythic thinking.

Susan Sontag, in *Illness as Metaphor*, aligns herself with this medical ideal in her crusade against metaphoric thinking about illness, which she sees as harmful and destructive. Though not literally a pathography, *Illness as Metaphor* is inspired by her personal experience of cancer. Ironically, the book participates in the very mythic thinking it criticizes. The myth of "metaphorlessness" is the organizing myth of *Illness as Metaphor*. This is the notion that illness can and should be experienced without recourse to metaphoric thinking, a functional myth that appears to help Sontag endure and recover from her illness. It is of interest that though she declares "that illness is *not* a metaphor, and that the most truthful way of regarding illness—and the healthiest way of being ill—is the one most purified of, most resistant to, metaphoric thinking," she introduces her book with an elaborate geographical metaphor comparing illness to a sojourn in a distant kingdom: "Illness is the night-side of life, a more onerous citizenship. Everyone who is born holds dual citizenship, in the kingdom of the well and in the kingdom of the sick. Although we all prefer to use only the good passport, sooner or later each of us is obliged, at least for a spell, to identify ourselves as citizens of that other place" (3).

The discrepancy here between precept and practice is important. For even if we agree with Sontag that illness should be stripped of metaphor, myth, and symbol—and not everyone will agree with her about this—it is an expectation that few of us could live up to.[11] Metaphoric thinking is built into our very mental faculties. Ironically, pathographers cite as helpful Sontag's metaphor of illness as the "kingdom of the sick" far more frequently than they do her idea that illness is best experienced without recourse to metaphoric thinking (Callen, 65; Creaturo, 92, 103; Schreiber, 70). As Robert Jay Lifton so aptly remarks, "We live on images. As human beings we know our bodies and our minds only through what we can imagine. To grasp our humanity we need to structure these images into metaphors and models" (1979, 3). Even Sontag realizes this, observing in *AIDS and Its Metaphors,* "Of course, one cannot think without metaphors" (5).

Pathography is invaluable to us as a way to study the metaphoric dimensions of the medical enterprise. Just to consider the titles of these books gives some indication of the metaphoric thinking that lies behind them: *Coming Back, Voyage and Return, Signs of Spring, Second Life, A Private Battle, Cancer Winner, Embracing the Wolf.* Not only does pathography restore the phenomenological and the experiential to the medical encounter, but it also restores the mythic dimension our scientific culture ignores or disallows.

Formulation

Pathography, then, provides us with a "taxonomy" of mythic attitudes about illness; it also helps us see just how a particular myth functions in a given situation. Sontag decries metaphoric thinking about illness because she focuses on its negative dimensions: for example, the myth that cancer is caused by "the repression of violent [or sexual] feelings," or that tuberculosis is "a disease of the soul" (1979, 22,17), or that AIDS is "a disease not only of sexual excess but of perversity" (1989, 26). What she fails to see in both her books is that myths about illness may be enabling as well as disabling: enabling, in that they can actually help the sick person who believes them to recover or, at least, to deal better with the circumstances of illness or death; disabling, in that they can impede a patient's ability to recover and even augment suffering. Pathography is a superb idiographic document because it shows us these myths and metaphors as they are "lived in"—for better or for worse.

In pathography, then, not only is mythic thinking pervasive, but it is functional—medically syntonic or dystonic, and personally enabling or disabling. But it is functional in a larger and deeper sense. The subject of these books is a kind of experience that is so painful, destructive, and disorienting that it results in a counterimpulse toward creation and order. This counterimpulse is what Lifton, in his celebrated study of the survivors of Hiroshima, calls "formulation," a reparative process that deals with trauma by imagination and interpretation. Formulation, Lifton remarks, is a kind of "psychic rebuilding," the construction of certain inner forms or configurations that function "as a bridge between self and world"—a psychological process whereby the individual suffering from trauma "returns" to the world of the living (1967, 367, 525–26). Formulation involves the effort to re-establish three elements essential to psychic function: the sense of connection (between self and other), the sense of symbolic integrity (seeing one's life as meaningful), and the sense of movement (the capacity for change) (367).[12] Lifton further describes the formulative process as "intimately bound up with mastery"; successful formulation "not only enhances mastery but, in an important sense, contains the mental representation of mastery" (536, 367). The act of formulation, then, involves the discovery of patterns in experience, the imposition of order, the creation of meaning—all with the purpose of mastering a traumatic experience and thereby re-establishing a sense of connectedness with objective reality and with other people. It is these things that enable human beings not only to live through severe illness or the death of a loved one but also to live beyond them.

Pathography can be seen as re-formulation of the experience of illness, as the artistic product and continuation of the instinctive psychological act of formulation: it gathers together the separate meanings, the moments of illumination and understanding, the cycles of hope and despair, and weaves them into a whole fabric, one wherein a temporal sequence of events takes on narrative form. Roy Pascal, describing autobiography, nicely sums up the narrative extension of this process of formulation: successful auto-biographies, he observes, "seem to suggest a certain power of the personality over circumstance, not in the arrogant sense that circumstance can be bent to the will of the individual, but in the sense that the individual can extract nurture out of disparate incidents and ultimately bind them together in his own way, disregarding all that was unusable. Painful as well as advantageous experiences can thus be transformed into the substance of the personality" (10–11). The psychological process of formulation as articulated by Lifton and the narrative act of reformulation embodied in pathography are in some sense parallel: both involve an individual's mastery of a set of circumstances, both suggest the act of constructing or piecing together a set of disparate events into a coherent whole, both concern the aesthetic act of seeing pattern and design and its epistemological analogue—the imposition of meaning or the discovery of significance.

Pathography can also be seen as the final stage in the process of formulation, completing the bridge between the suffering self and the outside world by an overt act of communication. Moreover, in pathography the need to *tell* others so often becomes the wish to *help* others: perhaps the movement from catharsis to altruism is a signal of the success of the formulation. As Bernice Kavinoky remarks of her pathography in a letter accompanying the manuscript: "This was a book that *had* to be written. I wrote it originally for myself, because it clarified my thinking and emotions. Then I began to ponder over it and felt perhaps it was for everybody—not only those who had my operation but everyone who had been through an experience of shock and loss, and who had eventually—after the flying of flags and lifting of the chin—to face it, in his own waiting room, alone" (71–72).

Myth in Pathography

Pathography is an immensely rich reservoir of the metaphors and models that surround illness in contemporary culture. These books are of value to us not because they record "what happened"—for they are not, as we have seen, factual accounts—but precisely because they *are* interpretations of experience. And as interpretations they must be understood as constructs, revisions, and, in some cases, creative distortions that expose a variety of ideological and mythic attitudes about illness today.

Many patient-authors will use a particular metaphor, mythic construct, or ideological paradigm to describe and explain their experience.[13] Quite often this central image functions as an organizational principle encompassing all aspects of an illness—disease, treatment, medical institutions and personnel. Some organizing myths are highly idiosyncratic. Thus Joanna Baumer Permut's pathography about lupus—the disease that takes its name from the Latin word for wolf—is shaped around her thoughts about the wolf. Each chapter is preceded by an epigram or quotation about wolves; each chapter title bears some reference to the wolf. The use of the name of the disease as an organizing metaphor seems successful in helping her come to terms with her condition. The pathography moves from an initial sense of victimization (the first chapter is titled, "The Wolf Stalks His Prey") to a final accommodation (the last chapter is called "Wolf and Patient Negotiate Peace"). As Permut observes, "the wolf image works for me. The metaphor serves the disease, and therefore my self positively" (163).

Eleanor Clark's pathography is also unusual in the choice of an organizing metaphor: the personal story of illness is set within the context of Homeric epic. Suffering from macular degeneration in both eyes, Clark spends her days writing her pathography and her evenings listening to readings of Homer's *Iliad* and *Odyssey,* an activity that she considers "inseparable from the rest of the story" (ix). She sees both epics—hers and Homer's—as similar in their concern with the theme of justice, and of course both are composed by a blind author. In general, though, the glorious world of Homer serves as a foil to which she contrasts the modern world, which she sees as deficient in heroism and lacking in any sense of death as meaningful. Clark's pathography is a very angry one, and the contrast she finds between the ancient and the modern serves as an apt expression of this anger.

A final example is Patricia Hingle's *A Coming of Roses,* intended primarily as an inspirational book for those who have (or will have) cancer. Life itself is the rose; cancer the thorn. Convinced that cancer has made her come to terms with the choices she has made in life, she begins her pathography with the words, "Cancer saved my life" (1). The metaphor is clearly an enabling one. The last chapter is titled "Regeneration": her rose garden has come into bloom, but, of course, the roses still have thorns. To Hingle, a rose garden in full bloom seems an apt metaphor for her condition, a rich and satisfying life in which her cancer is in remission.

But it would be a misnomer to call Permut's wolf or Clark's Homeric allusions or Hingle's rose garden "myths." Though they touch on mythic issues—the threat of the bestial other, the image of heroic excellence, and natural cycles of loss and renewal—they are really closer to elaborate metaphors in being conscious, artful, and "literary." In contrast, the mythic paradigms one finds in most contemporary pathographies seem at once more conventional and more "archetypal."

What is striking about pathography is the extent to which these very personal accounts of illness, though highly individualized, tend to be confined to certain repeated themes—themes of an archetypal, mythic nature. Over and over again, the same metaphorical paradigms are repeated in pathographies: the paradigm of regeneration, the idea of illness as 'battle, the athletic ideal, the journey into a distant country, and the mythos of healthy-mindedness. Why should the same paradigms recur with such frequency in pathography? George Rousseau notes that although "patients in Shakespeare's England will not describe themselves like those in Proust's Paris or Schnitzler's Vienna," nevertheless "similarities do appear: categories of thought so consistent in their metaphoric coherence (the patient as hero, disease as predatory invader-villain . . .)—so coherent that one wonders if there could be a heritage of myths about suffering in the Jungian archetypal sense" (169). The reader of pathographies must attend to both these differences and these similarities. It is not surprising that certain significant motifs and patterns—especially those concerned with phenomena that all human beings experience, such as growth and change or suffering, illness, and death—should recur over and over in very different periods and cultures. But it also makes sense that these deep-lying patterns should emerge in forms that are culturally inflected, shaped by a particular place and time. If pathography is an imaginative reformulation of experience that reconnects the isolated individual sufferer with his or her world, the connecting "formula" needs to be both culture-specific and transcultural, for the patient's world includes both a particular society at a certain moment in history and the larger and more timeless human community that underlies it.

Occasionally, the mythic and metaphoric themes one finds in pathography are overt and carefully elaborated. This is especially the case when the pathographer is a professional writer, with a writer's self-conscious concern for artistic craft and form. More often, though, the patterns are tacit and instinctive, surfacing in such isolated and unselfconscious phrases as "my battle with cancer" or "my journey to recovery." To the literary critic such paradigms may at first appear less interesting because they are so rarely artistically developed and because they are so often latent rather than overt. Indeed in some pathographies, the signifier almost disappears because the signified operates at so instinctive a level, resonating with deep, transpersonal images and patterns of meaning. The "fight with cancer" may be a throwaway phrase, casual and conventional, but it may also signal a way of dealing with illness that remains inarticulate because it is so profound: for such a patient or pathographer, sickness actually becomes a form of war. For the social critic, then, it is precisely the lack of literary sophistication and conscious development of such patterns that marks them as mythic and, thus, of interest.

For the literary critic, however, it is the richer and more elaborated pathography that best repays critical analysis. As one might expect, pathographies differ greatly in quality, ranging from sincere though unsophisticated works published by small denominational presses to profound literary explorations of illness and death such as John Donne's seventeenth-century *Devotions Upon Emergent Occasions* or Peter Noll's modern *In the Face of Death*. Importantly, Donne and Noll are individuals with an impressive range of intellectual and spiritual commitments as well as experienced writers. It is not accidental that the pathography offering the fullest and most imaginative version of the journey myth is authored by a skilled writer, Oliver Sacks. This is true of the military myth, too, where the pathographies that best deploy the myth with depth and insight are the work of professionals—Cornelius Ryan and Paul Monette.

Each of the mythic paradigms I have found repeated in pathography—battle, journey, rebirth, and "healthy-mindedness"—will be analyzed and explored in the chapters that follow. Division among them is inevitably arbitrary to some degree: the patient who experiences illness as a form of death and rebirth, for example, may also see it as a quest for a renewed life. Such blending is natural to myth and inevitable in literary works that evolve from it: to cite only one example, the *Aeneid* combines motifs of quest, regeneration, and war. In pathographies, too, there is necessarily some overlap between one mythic paradigm and another. But these paradigms must also be seen as disjunct: the myths do not organize themselves into any necessary or logical sequence. Consequently the chapters that analyze them can have no "through line" of developing argument. Such a unifying metamyth would exemplify mythic thinking at its most factitious, imposing pattern where it does not exist.

Nevertheless, the final discussion of healthy-mindedness provides a kind of closure and at the same time a significant reversal to the earlier chapters. Unlike the other myths to be considered, healthy-mindedness is not obviously archetypal; indeed, it is not really a narrative pattern at all. It is for this reason that I refer to this constellation of mythic ideas and values as "mythos" rather than "myth." Furthermore, whereas the myths of battle, journey, and rebirth inform the way individuals *understand* their illness, healthy-mindedness concerns not just the epistemological but also the pragmatic and the practical. I use the term to refer to a congeries of attitudes, assumptions, and practices that emerge in recent pathographies and that challenge the corresponding assumptions and practices of orthodox medicine.

Healthy-mindedness at every point differentiates itself from the scientism of the biomedical model: in its reliance on nature rather than *techné,* its appeal to anecdotal rather than statistical evidence, and its basis in a logic of symbols rather than the scientific logic of testing and experiment. It is thus not surprising that the therapies it offers often approximate mythical ways of thinking and behaving: to see love as the source of all healing borders on the religious; to give oneself injections of a substance made from red ants because these insects are "incredibly quick at bringing dead matter back into the life cycle" verges on the magical (Siegel and Melton; Chester, 133). The mythic dimension of healthy-mindedness is evident in both its contrast to science and its affiliations with other forms of mythic thought. It is a cultural myth—that is, a constellation of beliefs, values, and practices—that attracts our allegiance not because it can be proved but because in our culture it is felt by many to be true to their experience of illness.

Given its mythic character and lack of any specific narrative pattern, it is not surprising that the mythos of healthy-mindedness subsumes many of the myths we have been examining. Though these myths tend to reappear in healthy-minded pathographies, it is with a striking difference. Myth, we have observed, is analogical and dynamic. In most pathography, mythic analogies tend to translate the literal facts of illness and therapy into metaphors and symbols. Such metaphors and symbols, however, tend to be absent from healthy-minded pathographies: here, metaphor is translated into fact, so that mythic paradigms surface as actual practices rather than heuristic devices. For example, in a pathography organized around the journey or the battle myth, the paradigm serves as a way of metaphorically understanding the process of an illness. In a healthy-minded pathography, however, the myth of journey or battle actually *becomes* the action—meaning turns to praxis. So an AIDS patient, traveling to Tijuana to buy an illegal drug, is caught up in a literal quest for the "elixir" that will cure AIDS. And patients who visualize their white blood cells as knights fighting and defeating the invading cancer are attempting to convert symbolism into therapy, figure into fact. The dynamic tendency of all mythic thinking here achieves its fullest realization, as the battle myth is consciously used as an actual therapeutic device. We see why healthy-minded pathographies have no need of imagery that transforms the medical into the mythic: here, at last, myth has become medicine.

CHAPTER TWO

The Myth of Rebirth and the Promise of Cure

Rebirth Narratives: Tradition and Transformation

One explanation for the popularity of pathographies today is simply that they provide "a good read." Pathographies are compelling because they describe dramatic human experience of real crisis: they appeal to us because they give shape to our deepest hopes and fears about such crises, and in so doing, they often draw upon profound archetypal dimensions of human experience. If this is so, one might wonder why it is that pathographies were not more in evidence in previous eras and cultures. Why is it that these books are so rarely found before the mid-twentieth century? One answer to this question is that such narratives do exist in earlier periods, but they exist in a different form. It is my belief that our contemporary pathographies have their closest counterparts in a kind of literature that at first must seem radically different: autobiographies describing religious conversion. Indeed, it almost seems as though pathography has replaced the conversion autobiography of earlier, more religious cultures.

It is of interest that these two kinds of autobiographical narrative seem to preclude each other in the eras where they occur most frequently. Thus in seventeenth-century England, when autobiographies describing religious conversion flourished, extant personal accounts of illness in book-length form are quite rare. When we do find an autobiographical account of physical illness in this period, it is deflected toward the primary cultural mode—that is, the spiritual dimension. Thus John Donne's *Devotions Upon Emergent Occasions* not only treats physical illness as a means for spiritual growth but also consistently interprets the physical dimension as a metaphor for the spiritual. In contrast, the popular literature of America in the last few decades includes a remarkable number of pathographies and comparatively few spiritual autobiographies. Of course, people today still do undergo religious conversion, and they do write about these experiences; but these books are rarely "best-sellers," like some pathographies.

Clearly, the popularity of these two confessional genres in their respective periods reflects the cultural relevance of the experiences described. Spiritual autobiography is an eminently suitable genre for a culture that sets a high premium on the status of the soul and devalues the body as, at best, a temporary and faulty vessel. Pathography, on the other hand, is appropriate to a more materialistic culture where the physical replaces the spiritual as a central concern, where the physician replaces the clergyman as the agent in the healing process, and where scientific laws replace religious dogma. The prominence of spiritual autobiography in the seventeenth century and pathography in the late twentieth century reflects not so much frequency of conversion or disease as it does the mind-set of each culture: the spiritual realities of sin, repentance, and deliverance were as central to individuals in seventeenth-century England and America as are the physical realities of illness and recovery or death today.[1]

However, it is not the differences between these two bodies of narrative but their similarities that concern me here. One such likeness is the fact that both genres are monothematic: the desire to get well dominates pathography in the same way that the desire to be saved dominates autobiographies of conversion. This single theme generally serves as a selective principle, the organizing "plot," either editing out events that do not bear directly on illness or conversion or else subsuming them under it. Another similarity is the way both kinds of autobiographical narrative enable readers who share—or may come to share—a similar experience to understand it better by providing an expressive language and an interpretive framework. And as a function of this, both genres seem to serve for their readers as models—models that not only articulate experience but also help determine it.

Both spiritual autobiographies and pathographies assume that the experiences they describe are universals. The assumption that either religious or illness experience is generalizable is responsible for the way both kinds of narrative seem to serve as paradigms. In the introductory chapter, I discussed the ways in which pathography can serve as a model that shapes experience for its author and for its reader as well. As we have seen, sometimes authors of such books will cite another pathography as influential in helping them arrive at an understanding of their own experience. More commonly, authors will state that their motive for writing the book is that it be of help to others undergoing a similar illness. So Eileen Radziunas writes her pathography specifically for those afflicted with lupus and other "imposter diseases" (xii–xiv), and H. C. Brown intends his book about the fear associated with chronic heart disease to function as "a mirror into which you can look and look until insight comes" (220). In the same way, one function of spiritual autobiography is to serve as a model for its readers. Thus seventeenth-century Thomas Halyburton, in his *Memoirs,* expresses the wish that, should his religious autobiography "ever fall into the hands of any other Christian, it may not prove unuseful to him, considering that the work of the Lord, in substance, is uniform and the same in all; and 'as face answereth to face in a glass' so does one Christian's experience answer to another's" (Starr, 14). Both genres, then, are assumed to be capable of "mirroring" another's experience.

Perhaps the most striking similarity between pathographies and autobiographies of conversion is that both, with their focus on extraordinary or traumatic experience, give special prominence to myths about personal change. The myth of rebirth, which is central to autobiographies about conversion, is also the organizing construct for a good many pathographies. It turns on the belief that one can undergo a process of transformation so profound as to constitute a kind of death to the "old self" and rebirth to a new and very different self.

This myth is remarkable for its pervasiveness—it appears in nearly every culture and every era—and for the plasticity that allows it to be adapted to such different cultural milieus. It is a myth that seems as old as mythic thinking itself. Its narrative form is found in the story of Osiris; its ritual form in the Eleusinian mysteries and the rites of Dionysius. Moreover, it informs much Greek drama. For example, the conversion of the Furies into the Eumenides at the end of Aeschylus' *Oresteia* summarizes the redemptive and transforming logic of the whole trilogy. We see a similar change in Sophocles' mysterious "translation" of Oedipus at the moment of his death, an apotheosis that reverses his rise and fall earlier in his career. The same pattern turns to savage irony in Euripides' dark fantasy of rebirth in the *Bacchae.* The myth emerges in epic, too, as Virgil recasts Odysseus' journey to the land of the dead in the form of Aeneas' descent into the underworld—a "rebirth" that releases him from his Trojan past and propels him into his Roman future. With the advent of Christianity, the myth of rebirth assumes a position at the very center of both faith and practice: the death and resurrection of Christ is the central kerygma of the Christian faith, a divine paradigm that each individual is expected to try to emulate through a spiritual death and rebirth in his or her own life.

One obvious and important function of the rebirth myth is to resolve anxieties about death: if the soul is immortal, then the death of the body can be interpreted as a "rebirth" into a new and very different life. A variant on the rebirth pattern are the rituals of initiation from one stage or condition of life to another: the adolescent dies to childhood and is reborn as a man or a woman; the king or priest dies to his ordinary status and is reborn as secular or spiritual leader. The myth of rebirth, however, is not an anthropological anachronism and is not restricted to Christianity: on the contrary, it remains very much alive in contemporary culture—particularly in our psychological understandings of human life as a series of developmental stages and our infatuation with therapies that promise personal transformation and offer techniques to facilitate it. The myth of rebirth is alive today because it works: it "satisfies" us in several ways. This myth serves as wish-fulfillment, providing assurance that if we find ourselves and our lives less than satisfactory, they can always be changed. It also accounts for our sense of incompletion: the rebirth myth is associated with the fantasy that some day we might awaken to the "real self"—that we might be restored to ourselves and recover fully from the existential malaise that seems endemic to the human condition in a fallen world.

In spiritual autobiography, the myth of rebirth is manifested in the theme of conversion;[2] in pathography, in the widespread assumption that a traumatic illness, particularly if it brings one close to death, can result in a sense of regeneration and renewal. As we will see, in both kinds of narrative the rebirth myth has two primary components: the notion that the self is somehow transformed and the impression that for this changed self the whole world appears new and different.

The conversion experience is most commonly the dramatic climax of a spiritual autobiography and is frequently described as an unforgettable, miraculous event, accompanied by voices, dazzling lights, and subsequent feelings of peace and tranquillity. The prototype of this kind of experience is the conversion of Paul on the road to Damascus, when he is suddenly and traumatically wrenched by supernatural intervention from one set of beliefs and practices to another. Saul, the persecutor of the early Church, finds himself surrounded by a heavenly light, whereupon he falls to the ground and hears a divine voice chide him, "Why persecutest thou me?" After three days without food, drink, or sight, he is "reborn" with a new name, a new faith, and a new life (Acts 9). Countless individuals thereafter have used the Pauline prototype as a model for their own religious conversions. Augustine in *The Confessions* recounts a conversion experience in the Pauline mode. He describes his early life as one of indulgence in the pleasures of mind and body, a "death" out of which he is suddenly and finally reborn: overhearing a child singing *"tolle lege, tolle lege"* (take up and read), he feels compelled to pick up and read a particular scriptural passage, and—in his own words—"instantly . . . it was as though the light of certainty flooded into my heart and all the darkness of doubt vanished" (8.12; translation mine). The advent of Protestantism introduced a somewhat different model of conversion, a more graduated process consistent with Calvinist and Lutheran ideas of regeneration as a lifelong process made up of a series of definite stages. Thus in John Bunyan's spiritual autobiography, *Grace Abounding to the Chief of Sinners,* the sudden, fulminant conversion of Paul and Augustine gives way to a series of dramatic turning points. One such experience—in fact it is the event that initiates his regeneration—demonstrates the influence of the Pauline model. During a forbidden Sabbath-day game, the voice of a displeased God suddenly darts from heaven into his soul, crying, "Wilt thou leave thy sins, and go to Heaven, or have thy sins and go to Hell?" Bunyan stands transfixed, "in the midst of my play, before all that then were present," as the seeds of his conversion are sown (12–13; syntax and spelling are modernized). Thomas Merton in the twentieth century makes similar claims in *The Seven Storey Mountain* to sudden moments of awakening to "a new world" and convictions that he had been "reborn" (210–11,113). Other accounts of dramatic conversions can be found in William James's classic study of religious conversion, *The Varieties of Religious Experience:* these include experiences of unearthly light, disembodied voices, sweet smells and tastes, heart palpitations, hovering angels—and they almost always conclude with the sense that the convert's life has been finally and irrevocably changed.[3]

Not only is rebirth also a common theme in pathography, but it is represented in such a way as to recall the conversion experiences of spiritual autobiography. For example, David Tate, a young man with stage IV Hodgkin's disease (at a time before this illness could be cured) describes a dramatic and sudden conversion-like experience that changes the entire course of his illness. Quite suddenly, while meditating on his condition, he hears a voice tell him it is imperative that he *know* with absolute certainty that he is already cured. His acceptance of this certainty initiates a remarkable recovery from his illness, as well as an equally remarkable transformation in personality and life-style. He writes: "When I left the study, I was a different person. I was no longer ill with cancer. My life was no longer threatened. I was cured. This was a fact, something I knew" (58). Tate's experience strongly resembles that of George Melton, who, in his pathography about AIDS, describes a "healing dream" that he considers a turning point: from this moment on, he feels certain that recovery will follow, and it does. Another pathographer for whom recovery appears as a kind of conversion is Mary Kay Blakely, who compares her feelings upon leaving the hospital after a nine-day coma to the happiness of "a born-again fundamentalist" and even refers to herself as "a reborn" (251, 257).

Narratives describing heart problems seem especially likely to be organized around the myth of rebirth; indeed, some are uncannily similar to spiritual autobiographies. Perhaps this has something to do with the fact that the part of the body affected is the heart, for centuries the seat of the soul, source of life, and emblem of love. Moreover, both forms of personal narrative center on a specific incident of crisis, a dramatic event that in both cases determines how these authors perceive their lives before the event and how they hope to change them afterwards. In pathography, the individual who survives a heart attack or heart surgery and who must subsequently change his or her pattern of living to accommodate and protect the weakened organ frequently experiences this change as renewal and rejuvenation. Philip Roth remarks, following an emergency five-vessel coronary bypass, that after the surgery "I felt reborn—at once reborn and as though I had given birth" (225). And Nyles Reinfeld, after his coronary bypass, explicitly compares himself to the contemporary "born-again" Christian (51).

James L. Johnson's pathography is a striking instance of the parallelism between pathographies about heart disease and autobiographies about conversion. In fact, his description of his four-vessel coronary bypass surgery seems at times surprisingly close to spiritual autobiography, as the title suggests—*Coming Back: One Man's Journey to the Edge of Eternity and Spiritual Rediscovery.* The critical turning point that causes Johnson to rethink the meaning of his life and the values by which he lives is a medical trauma that brings him close to death. He comes to believe that "my confrontation with death was God's way of opening up a whole new world of spiritual rediscovery" (Prologue). Though Johnson had already been converted years before, he describes his recovery as others have described their conversions. Thus the ordinary world to which he "returns" after his symbolic journey into a different realm seems brighter and newer; he feels as though he is seeing familiar objects for the first time (94, 115). And when he returns home after surgery for a long convalescence, he feels he has been given "a new vision of life and myself at last" (122). As in autobiographies about religious conversion, Johnson undergoes a kind of transformation from one set of values and behaviors to another. Forced by his illness from a life of hyperactivity into what he calls an "enforced sabbatical," he observes that the "slowed-down pace was beginning to rebuild something within me that had been missing for so long" (122).

In both spiritual autobiography and pathographies about heart disease, the dramatic focal episode of a spiritual crisis or a coronary event has an impact on the author's sense of the "shape" of his or her life. In both kinds of narrative, the experience serves as a turning point around which authors retrospectively interpret their lives before the crisis and prospectively plan the life that lies ahead. Though in both cases the narrative structure tends to parallel the perceived shape of the experience, the way in which this is accomplished differs. In conversion narratives, the literary structure is usually tripartite: life-before-conversion, conversion itself, life-after-conversion. The life preceding a religious conversion is described as one of great sinfulness, the conversion itself is recounted in minute detail, and the life following conversion is conceived as one wherein the convert struggles to conform behavior and thoughts to what is believed to be the will of God. This is the dominant pattern in autobiographies describing conversion from the *Confessions* of Augustine in the fourth century to *The Seven Storey Mountain* of Thomas Merton in the twentieth.

Pathographical descriptions of cardiac disease also imply this tripartite structure, but it is retrospective, not sequential. Thus these narratives often begin in the coronary intensive care unit where the authors, recovering from their heart attacks or from the heart surgery that often follows a coronary, describe the crisis that sent them there and then reflect upon their lives. As the past is reconstructed in such a way as to make the heart attack intelligible, retrospectively "expected," and thus less threatening,[4] these authors invariably come to the realization that they ate too much, smoked too often, exercised too little, and were under a great deal of stress. The latter part of the narrative usually refers to the author's plan to adopt a new life-style and sometimes extends itself into his or her actual attempts to do so.

This way of shaping one's life retrospectively usually accompanies a certain conception of the self. In both pathography and conversion narratives, authors interpret their former lives from the vantage point of the conversion experience or the heart attack: they reevaluate everything they did and were in terms of that cataclysmic and definitive event. This establishes a felt distance not only from the former life but also from the former self. In seventeenth-century spiritual autobiography, the convention by which this is accomplished is to describe oneself as "chief of sinners"—a distinction routinely claimed by converts in their writings. So John Bunyan entitles his spiritual autobiography *Grace Abounding to the Chief of Sinners*, and Oliver Cromwell writes that before his conversion, "I lived in and loved darkness, and hated light; I was a chief, the chief of sinners."[5] It is not only the male sinner who feels he has earned this distinction: the Baptist Anna Trapnel also calls herself the "chief of sinners" in her autobiography, and Sarah Wright is similarly entitled in a narrative of her life by Henry Jessey (Tindall, 30, 37).

The corresponding term in twentieth-century pathography is the "type A personality," described in one contemporary book on heart disease as a complex of personality traits including "excessive competitive drive," "aggressive impatience," and "a sense of time urgency or 'hurry sickness'" (Friedman, 51–79). The authors of pathographies about cardiac disease repeatedly perceive and describe themselves as "type A personalities"; sometimes as "coronary-prone personalities." Just as religious converts tend to perceive in their former lives only sinfulness—and may even exaggerate their faults in order to present a more satisfying portrait of themselves as utterly depraved—so perhaps heart attack victims tend to perceive in their character precisely those traits that comprise the type A personality.

The two terms are analogous not only in their meaning but also in their function: both in a subtle way are self-congratulatory. For converts to see themselves in their former lives as "chief of sinners" seems itself a kind of self-aggrandizement, particularly since the actual sins enumerated always seem somewhat trivial. Bunyan excoriates himself in his autobiography as follows: "I was more loathsome in my own eyes than was a toad, and I thought I was so in God's eyes too. . . . I thought none but the Devil himself could equal me for inward wickedness and pollution of mind" (29; spelling modernized). What he has actually *done* to merit this kind of self-characterization is to harbor blasphemous thoughts, swear, and play games on the Sabbath. This habit of exaggerated self-deprecation serves the larger religious values of a theocentric culture, since the greater the depravity of the sinner, the more glory to God in the sinner's conversion.

Pathographies about heart disease function in a similar though not identical way. Perceiving oneself as a "type A personality" or as "coronary-prone" is also self-congratulatory, since it castigates the self for precisely those traits that our culture values most—aggressiveness, competitiveness, the wish to achieve, and the ability to do so. Thus one pathographer characterizes himself before heart surgery as aggressive, competitive, and extroverted, remarking that cardiac disease destroys his "myth of super-competence" (Mandell, 46). It is not at all uncommon for the individual who characterizes him or herself as a type A personality to use those same behavior patterns and attitudes in the very attempt to "convert" to a type B personality. And it is, in fact, a kind of conversion. Not only must these type A heart patients change their outer behavior—give up smoking, lose weight, avoid certain foods—but they are expected to change their very characters. The older model of conversion here fits perfectly, in its insistence that a *conversio mori* (change of habits) must be accompanied by a *conversio mentis* (change of mind).

The majority of pathographies about heart disease describe this shift in character and life-style, though they vary greatly in the style with which they do so. Some are floridly metaphoric: James L. Johnson observes that "as a 'type A' personality my radiator ran hot all the time" and remarks of his angiogram, "God was blowing the whistle on me, trying to get my attention" (13, 34). Some tend toward the prosaic: Bea Keiser comments on the way her husband's heart attack "forced our family to re-examine our life-style and offered us a fuller and enriched family structure" (Introduction). Some prefer a quasi-scientific approach: Arnold Mandell, using the concepts and terminology of neuroscience, represents the change in character he hopes to effect as a transition from "the first-cycle issues of the middle-brain" to the more "spiritual" upper-brain, and the desired change in behavior as a movement from an extroverted life of aggressiveness and competitiveness to one of inwardness, contemplativeness, and detachment (15–34).[6]

As a functional myth, the concept of rebirth operates in both kinds of autobiography in parallel ways: it enables these authors to perceive their sickness, whether spiritual or physical, as the obvious outcome of a particular life-style or personality type, giving them the impetus to change their lives in the desired direction. Cardiac arrest or a sudden conversion experience thus precipitates a dramatic change from one set of values to another and a concomitant transformation in life-style.

The reader is not as likely to find the rebirth myth foregrounded in pathographies about cancer, perhaps because cancer, unlike heart attack, is not primarily organized around acute episodes. Because of the nature of the disease, a cancer patient does not find that "the date of rebirth and revitalization can be fixed accurately," as one pathographer with heart disease observed of his bypass surgery (Reinfeld, 51). But the analogy between pathography and spiritual autobiography still holds in regard to illnesses like cancer, since not all spiritual autobiographies are organized around acute episodes either. Besides the Pauline conversion model—that sudden, dramatic moment of regeneration—there is the more gradual "lysis" conversion described by James as characteristic of the conversions of Bunyan and Tolstoy—a gradual process of unification proceeding in a series of graduated stages (152). Whereas the dramatic sense of regeneration and renewal that can follow a heart attack is most similar to "crisis" conversions of the Pauline type, the experience of recovery from cancer, with its remissions and relapses, is more like the "lysis" conversion model.

Again we find the author's depiction of him or herself in pathography as conforming to a certain personality type—in this case, the "cancer-prone personality."[7] This myth of self functions for the cancer patient in the same way that the idea of the "type A personality" does for the heart patient: it makes a correlation between exterior, physical symptoms and an interior, psychological or spiritual condition; it satisfies the need to find a cause for the illness; and it suggests a basis for cure in simply eliminating the causal agent.

Some individuals with cancer are much less happy with the notion of a "type C personality" than are individuals who have heart disease with their label. Susan Sontag is a vociferous opponent of the idea that cancer is associated with psychological traits. She sees such psychologizing as destructive because it "undermines the 'reality' of a disease" and because it seems "to provide control over the experiences and events (like grave illnesses) over which people have in fact little or no control" (1979, 54). However, a fair number of cancer patients, particularly those who use visualization therapy, find undermining the "reality" of their disease to be helpful, and Sontag's assumption that sick people have no control over their illnesses is one that many pathographers would challenge.

The functional similarity between the "chief of sinners" and the "type A personality" or the "cancer-prone personality" suggests that the contemporary habit of associating psychological qualities with illness may be analogous to (if not derived from) the older association between sin and disease. Though physical illness today is considered a biochemical phenomenon, people often experience their illnesses as intrinsically linked with interior qualities of psyche and spirit, for good or for ill: the "signs" of an illness are thought to signify an interior mental or spiritual condition. Medieval and Renaissance thinking commonly understood physical illness as evidence of a diseased spiritual condition. According to the anonymous author of a fifteenth-century tract on the art of dying, "bodily sickness cometh of the sickness of the soul" (Beaty, 27). Two centuries later, John Donne observes that "sin is the root and the fuel of all sickness" (148), while the Anglican divine Jeremy Taylor counsels the ill person to "use [illness] as a punishment for thy sins, and so God intends it" (79). The association between sin and disease is usually denounced today as an atavistic superstition that only serves to victimize further the ill person.[8] However, this myth has the capacity to be enabling as well as disabling. It is not always, as critics like Sontag imply, a myth imposed on the ill by a superstitious, ignorant, or malicious public but is sometimes actively embraced by patients themselves.

One example of a cancer patient who identifies with a certain personality type is Anthony Sattilaro, himself a physician, who believes that his cancer is the product of "my many years of selfishness, my overpowering drive for self-gratification, and my unwillingness to see others as anything but competitors" (201). What is striking about this "confession" of sins that lead to cancer is that it actually *is* just that: Sattilaro is here describing what he says to a priest during the Roman Catholic rite of confession. On another occasion, when he is giving a talk on cancer and macrobiotics, Sattilaro makes a similar admission, a secular "confession" that recalls the public recital of faith formerly required for admittance to some Protestant denominations: "I had lived a life of selfishness, greed, self-centered ambition, and fear. I was bent on satisfying my own appetites, and was intractable in my dealings with others. I viewed life as a dog-eat-dog existence; it was the contest of getting what one could for one's self, and the hell with the rest of the world." He allows that a bad diet was the direct cause of his cancer but insists that it was those personality traits "that created the person who was attracted to such a regimen as mine." Sattilaro concludes with a declaration of the age-old equation between sin and disease: "This clutching for pleasures of the senses, and for material possessions, is what gives rise to cancer, I believe" (207). Accompanying his self-castigation for what he sees as the spiritual defects of "the paragon cancer victim"—and maybe, in part, because of this—Sattilaro experiences a conversion-like awakening of his "intuitive nature": "I went from focusing my attention on viruses and cells under a microscope to sitting back and contemplating the vast interwoven mosaic of the universe" (178). "Conversion" coincides with cure: the last sentence of the book announces with finality, "I was diagnosed by my physicians as in 'complete remission'" (Epilogue).

Many pathographers, like Sattilaro, report illness to be an occasion for spiritual growth. In *The Glory Woods,* Virginia Greer describes cancer as "without a doubt the most awesome experience of my life," one that, she feels, brings her closer to God (137). Anne Hargrove uses language reminiscent of spiritual autobiography to describe her feeling of renewal: "The experience of having cancer is turning me into a new creature. I have chosen to exchange the ways of death for a new life and have felt the stirrings of a new creature within me, myself newly conceived" (44). This way of describing the sense of personal or spiritual growth is not restricted to pathographies about cancer. We have seen how James L. Johnson credits the bypass surgery that brings him close to death as "God's way of opening up a whole new world of spiritual rediscovery" (Prologue). Laura Chester, in her pathography about lupus, writes that "illness can almost be seen as an opportunity" for rediscovering "the spiritual world" (74). Surprisingly, even a perceived recovery from AIDS can elicit this kind of thinking: George Melton, in a chapter of his pathography called "My Awakening," sees AIDS as "a message from my body," alerting him to the need for a more spiritually centered sense of life (54).

Illness often serves as an occasion not only for personal growth but also for dramatic personal change. Heart attack victims, as we have seen, regularly describe the change to a slower, less stressful, and more meditative style of life. Serious illness of all kinds usually results in an enforced period of passivity—a "time-apart" during which values of self and society can be questioned and, sometimes, new values asserted in their place. Often the hospital setting, especially if it includes time spent in an intensive care unit, serves as the locus for this hiatus in the course of a life. What for some is experienced as the senseless interruption of a life of purpose and meaning is for others an unexpected opportunity to stand back and evaluate that life.

Mary Kay Blakely, a hassled, overwrought mother and journalist who suddenly goes into a nine-day coma, finds that such an experience compels her, and others too, "to stop and think, to abandon the mindless path of the starving processionaries" (262). This "mindless path" is Blakely's elliptical term for a life-style that is pressured, stressful, and success-oriented; the "good" she finds is a new perspective on life that enables her to see the difference between personal and societal goals. This understanding is itself a kind of "rebirth"—a birth of the newly individuated self, perceived as radically distinct from the needs and pressures of the society to which it belongs. Blakely leaves the hospital with a very different perspective on her life: "After awakening . . . I gradually discovered that the life planned by the woman I had been no longer fit the woman I'd become" (261).

Like all cultural myths, however, the notion of illness as a form of rebirth or an occasion for spiritual growth is, for some people, disabling. This notion surfaces as a kind of antimyth in Stephanie Cook's pathography, where extensive and mutilating treatments for choriocarcinoma are followed by her return to ordinary life with the sense of it as a "diminished thing." Describing her "poisonous impatience with normality," she remarks that during her illness "I had been reduced to some highly concentrated essence of myself. I was beginning to suspect that nothing ever again would be as real to me as the cancer had been" (260). One wonders if the title of this book, *Second Life,* is not an ironic comment on the reversal she has experienced of the myth of rebirth. A somewhat different example is Fitzhugh Mullan's *Vital Signs,* where the expected sense of renewal after surviving a life-threatening illness does not materialize. Mullan suffers not only the surgical removal of a tumor in his chest but also a second, unanticipated thoracotomy (a surgical incision of the chest wall) as a result of the accidental severing of a vein during an early biopsy. After such drastic procedures, he anticipates being a "different person" (103). But he is bitterly disappointed: "I had come so close to death that I imagined my perspective on life would be different. I fantasized that certain personal pettinesses of mine would disappear and that I would be wiser and more temperate than I had been before. . . . much to my dismay, things were not different. . . . My personality . . . was definitely not 'born again'" (103–4).

That this myth can generate complaints of its ineffectiveness or its unhelpfulness is actually a sign of its vitality. The mark of a living myth is not so much its veracity, nor even its utility—for all cultural myths are capable of being at times enabling or disabling—but its authority and power, the degree to which people feel compelled to believe in it. An essay by the late Anatole Broyard in the *New York Times Magazine* (Nov. 12, 1989) and the strong reactions this essay excited effectively illustrate the power of this myth—for good or for ill. Broyard's article, "Intoxicated by My Illness," is a brief but beautifully written description of the heightening of awareness he experiences during his cancer experience. Despite the pain and indignity he suffers, his primary response to his illness is one of "elation" and "intoxication." Thus he describes with great eloquence the sense that his body has been "reborn as a brand-new infatuation" and "the rich sense of crisis" that restores to ordinary reality its miraculous nature. Responses to Broyard's brief pathography range from delighted recognition to angry resentment. The author of one letter recalls her own illness with its "months of mental imaging and heightened spirituality"; another remembers with obvious pleasure how her "liberation, through illness, to the world of nature and of beauty, of poetry and music" helped her survive a cancer experience. A third letter, however, attacks the idea that illness is "a path to growth through adversity"; such an intimidating ideal, argues the author, is likely to set an "unreasonable model" for the ordinary cancer patient and to elicit unsympathetic reactions from family and friends when the patient fails to "measure up." [9]

The power of a myth is also reflected in the various forms, symbols, and analogies it generates. The rebirth myth occurs most frequently as a sense of inner renewal and a feeling of spiritual growth—impressions illustrated in the pathographies described above. Another form the rebirth myth can take in pathography is suggested by metaphors from nature. And the world of nature, with its cycles of renewal in the springtime, seems indeed an apt representation of the feelings of regeneration that can accompany a serious illness.

Several pathographies use some metaphor from nature as their organizing construct. Laurel Lee's *Signs of Spring* is a journal begun while in remission from Hodgkin's disease; continued during the months of surgery, chemotherapy, and radiation that attend upon the return of her cancer; and concluded when she again goes into remission. As the title of her pathography implies, the revitalization of the natural world after the bleakness of winter seems especially appropriate to a cancer experience, where remission, with its promise of life renewed, seems very much like a rebirth. The analogy between physical and seasonal "rebirth" is given concrete form here as the author describes, at the end of her pathography, the garden she plants—a hopeful metaphor for her physical state. The use of a metaphor from nature is also central to Patricia Hingle's *A Coming of Roses*. This pathography, as we have seen, is organized around the analogy between cancer and the rose: life becomes the flower, and cancer, the thorns. The last chapter is very similar to the conclusion of *Signs of Spring:* entitled "Regeneration," it refers to the flowering of Hingle's rose garden and, by analogy, to her physical condition as a cancer patient in remission. But it is not only a cancer remission that can suggest an analogy with the regeneration of living things in the spring. Near the end of his pathography about AIDS, in a chapter called "My Awakening"—written as winter gives way to spring— George Melton observes: "From within my own being the new shoots of my true reality were beginning to push through the surface of a seemingly deteriorating body. For the first time the season seemed to affirm back to me the inevitability of my own rebirth" (46).

Doris Schwerin's *Diary of a Pigeon Watcher* is of especial interest because the pathography's formulation—a metaphor drawn from nature—substitutes for the author's expectation that feelings of heightened consciousness and deep personal transformation will follow upon an episode of serious illness. Recovering from a radical mastectomy, Schwerin anticipates "instant purification . . . a change in me, a feeling of blessedness for each moment" (9). These quasi-spiritual expectations never materialize, however, and she is painfully disappointed that such feelings of insight and renewal have not come to pass. As she tries to deal with her anger and confusion, she happens to notice some pigeons nesting on a ledge outside her New York City apartment window. She becomes interested in their lives, and this interest turns into an absorbing activity that sustains her through the five-year interval required for her remission to be called a cure. The pathography is, in effect, organized around the lives of these pigeons: watching them is the occasion for her to reflect on her own past—her "nest," as she calls it—and the pigeons' cycles of birth and maturation, extending over a five-year period, are a visible and compelling reminder of her hoped-for renewal.

A remarkable and highly unusual pathography is Terry Tempest Williams's *Refuge*, a book that uses nature metaphor as its organizing construct, but without the overtones of renewal and rebirth so typical of most pathographies of this kind. The author, a thirty-four-year-old Mormon and a naturalist, situates her mother's five-year illness and death from ovarian cancer within the overarching story of the rising of the Great Salt Lake in Utah during the same period and its devastating effect on the Bear River Migratory Bird Refuge, flooded for years. Each chapter bears the name of one of the birds associated with the Refuge; each chapter is preceded by a measurement of the lake level as it gradually rises.

In one sense, the pathography's formulation is the analogy between her mother's fatal illness and the gradual devastation of the Bird Refuge from the rising waters of the lake, which technology fails to control. This formulation organizes the emotion-laden events in a mother's long illness and painful death within a cycle of nature that in itself is value-free. In another sense, the Bird Refuge, "devastated by the flood, now begin[ning] to heal" in 1990, as she completes the book, represents the author herself, recovering from her mother's death: "Volunteers are beginning to reconstruct the marshes just as I am trying to reconstruct my life" (3). Exploring these analogies in writing the book enables the author to come to terms with her mother's death: "I have been in retreat," she writes. "This is my return" (4).

This formulation seems to be the product of Williams's deliberate rejection of the more common myth of war that surrounds cancer treatment today. Accompanying her mother for her first chemotherapy treatment, the author muses on the way "medical language is loaded . . . with military metaphors: the fight, the battle, enemy infiltration, and defense strategies." She wonders whether "this kind of aggression waged against our own bodies is counterproductive to healing" and asks, "how can we rethink cancer?" (43). Her response to this question is grounded in her recognition that the cancer process is similar to the creative process: though cancer is often viewed as an external, foreign, reified entity, in fact it originates within one's own body, slowly and invisibly growing, just as ideas are born and develop within the recesses of the unconscious mind. Her realization of the continuity between her mother's body and the land, and her perception of the embeddedness of human life within the cycle of nature are consistent with her identity as a woman, as a naturalist, and as a Mormon with deep ties to the land of her people.

Given the depth and extent of the formulating myth in this pathography—and the comfort afforded by the continuity the author perceives between human life and the world of nature—the book's ending comes as a surprise. The chapter-length epilogue continues the formulating myth of the continuity between the human and the natural, but for a very different purpose. Entitled "The Clan of the One-Breasted Women" (all previous chapters have taken their titles from the names of birds), the epilogue chronicles the many women in her family (including the author) who have been treated for or died from breast cancer. Unlike the story of her mother's death, these encounters with cancer are not accepted as a part of the cycles of nature but are attributed directly to radiation from above-ground atomic testing in a site in Nevada deemed "virtually uninhabited desert terrain," from 1951 to 1962: "my family and the birds at Great Salt Lake were some of the 'virtual uninhabitants'" (287). It is only at this point that the reader fully understands the book's complete title: *Refuge: An Unnatural History of Family and Place*. It is ironic that the military way of thinking that she repudiates early on as a metaphor should return here as a literal and destructive reality. Given our eagerness to create and deploy potentially dangerous technology in all areas of our culture—the military, the medical, the industrial—this irony gives added force to the need she perceives for us to reconceive the way we understand a disease like cancer and its treatments.

The Religious Formulation: Donne's *Devotions* and Contemporary Religious Pathographies

Death-and-resurrection is the central doctrine of the Christian faith and, therefore, it may seem surprising that my discussion of the rebirth myth, with its themes of regeneration and spiritual growth, has so far included no overtly religious pathographies—with the sole exception of James L. Johnson's *Coming Back*. One reason is that those narratives tend to be overshadowed by their secular counterparts: though they do exist, they seem to be published by small denominational presses and thus tend to have a smaller and narrower readership. Of those pathographies where the authors identify themselves as believing and practicing a particular religious faith,[10] a good many tend to avoid all mythic and metaphoric constructs—including the religious.

In Peter Paul Michael's *Multiple Sclerosis: A Dragon with a Hundred Heads*, the only evidence of metaphor is in the subtitle, though he is a Roman Catholic whose religion is clearly helpful in coming to terms with illness. Helen Hostetler's *A Time to Love*, a pathography written by a Mennonite about her son's illness and death from AIDS, though it is tesellated with biblical quotations, is similarly lacking in the rich use of metaphor and myth that we find in so many other pathographies. More commonly, religion enters these pathographies allusively: authors remember that they prayed just before or just after an operation; they mention friends and church groups who met and prayed together for their recovery; they engage in religious plea-bargaining, promising God some act of charity (often the pathography itself) if their lives are spared; or they choose a title with religious overtones, such as *Walking through the Fire*, a title taken from the Old Testament book of Isaiah, or *A Time to Love*, an allusion to the Old Testament book of Ecclesiastes.

It is possible that individuals with strong religious beliefs simply do not need to write pathographies. In my introductory chapter, I have argued that pathography derives from the need to find meaning in an illness experience. For the individual with firm religious convictions, the inherent meaningfulness of his or her suffering is assumed from the beginning. The Christian understanding of sin and redemption, for example, endows individual suffering with purpose and significance. Indeed, the very fact that sickness occurs in the context of a purposive universe and a loving deity makes it meaningful. Perhaps this is the reason why pathographies whose organizing construct is religious are not more plentiful and prominent: the individual's faith replaces the need for such a narrative formulation.

The pathographies I have read imply that orthodox Christianity today no longer occupies the position of ideological centrality that it held in earlier centuries. To compare these pathographies to Donne's *Devotions* suggests the degree to which religion in our time—even for believers—may have lost some of its imaginative centrality and interpretive power. An instructive illustration of this is *Comeback*, a pathography written by a born-again Christian who is a pitcher for a major league baseball team. When Dave Dravecky submits to surgery to remove a tumor on his pitching arm, his doctors assure him that he will never play again. But he does return to the pitcher's mound, to the amazement of his physicians, in a "comeback" that is applauded by thousands of cheering fans. The authenticity of this man's faith is unquestionable, and yet it does not really shape his pathography: the organizing construct for this book—its formulation—is baseball, not religion.[11]

Athletic pathographies like Dravecky's form a popular subdivision of the genre, and we shall examine some in the next chapter. However, the mythos that threatens to displace religion in our times is not sports, but science. "I trust Denton Cooley and the Lord," asserts a Baptist minister who undergoes open-heart surgery to replace his mitral and aortic valves (Brown, 141). This confession of faith establishes priorities that are probably instinctive and most certainly unselfconscious: God is assigned a role, but Denton Cooley, the surgeon, gets top billing. The fact that even a clergyman instinctively gives his physician precedence over God would seem to emphasize the displacement of religion in contemporary pathography and exemplifies the pervasive tendency to displace the divine, the diabolic, and the afterlife with constructs (and agents) of science and technology. A similar pathography in this respect is Kenneth Shapiro's *Dying and Living: One Man's Life with Cancer.* Told on three separate occasions that death is imminent, this man attributes his near-miraculous survival to his doctors and their treatment, himself, and God—in random order (117). He observes that "the patient *must* believe in his or her treatment . . . in order for it to work" and further remarks, "I had become a believer in immunotherapy"—indeed, he asserts that he believes in the human immunological system as "the answer to every disease in the world" (53). Shapiro's language, with its insistence on the word "believe," suggests the degree to which religious habits of thought continue to color attitudes toward illness.

But therapies are not appropriate objects of belief nor are doctors divine healers. There is danger in endowing the secular and the human with the qualities of the divine and in the expectations that result from this habit. When one pathographer is told by his doctor that he needs a second operation for his heart condition, the news comes as a shock: "Somehow I was convinced he should have pulled some miracle drug out of his sleeve" (Reinfeld, 45). The clichés here are not just clichés; medicine *is* expected to work miracles, and the doctor too often is regarded as a kind of magician, if not a deity.

Thus we have come full circle. Even if science has tended to replace religion as the official mythology of a secular culture, religious ways of thinking and imagining still persist, as if from a deeper instinctive level and an earlier age. If this is so, then we might expect the myth of rebirth to be especially well delineated in those contemporary pathographies—however few they may be—where religion is the author's organizing construct. Surprisingly, this turns out not to be so. In order to understand why, it may be helpful—before we analyze these pathographies—to turn back the cultural clock and scrutinize a religious pathography from an earlier era than our own.

John Donne's *Devotions Upon Emergent Occasions* is a rare example of a pathography composed in premodern times—written, moreover, during the flowering of spiritual autobiography; it is also a superbly crafted literary work, still capable, even in our secular age, of eliciting powerful emotional responses from its reader. The subject and purpose of the *Devotions* is as much the glorification of God as the understanding of an illness; nonetheless, the actual structure of the work (and the theme of each separate devotion) is based upon the medical facts of Donne's disease, which is typhus. The narrative begins with the premonitory signs of illness and subsequent "taking to the sick-bed." The physician is sent for; he arrives, is uncertain of what is wrong, and sends for more physicians, one of whom is the king's own private doctor. Therapy at first consists of giving cordials to protect the heart from "the venom and the malignity of the disease" (69) and laying pigeons at the feet to draw malignant vapours downwards. Finally the sickness "declares itself" by symptomatic spots. Donne then enters upon the seven "critical days" of his illness. When he shows signs of making a recovery, the physicians proceed with purgatives. The book ends with Donne cured but fearful of a relapse.

The organizing construct that explains the meaning both of the illness itself and of the various treatments to which Donne is subjected is religious belief. In accord with an underlying sacramentalism, all physical realities have a spiritual dimension and a spiritual analogue: illness is thus inherently meaningful and purposive. Not only is the physical dimension consistently interpreted as a metaphor for the spiritual, but physical realities are always subordinated to their spiritual counterparts. What is most important is the condition of the soul, not the body, and illness serves as a visible sign of an underlying and invisible spiritual condition. "I know that in the state of my body," writes Donne, "which is more discernible than that of my soul, thou dost effigiate my soul to me" (50). Physical signs thus serve as diagnostic indicators of a spiritual malaise, so that when Donne's illness "declares itself" by the appearance of spots on the chest, he likens these to the spots of sin on the soul. The absence of such symptoms suggests sins that are hidden and secret and therefore doubly dangerous, whereas their appearance reveals the nature of the illness and thus indicates to physicians—of body or of soul—how they should proceed. Treatment, then, depends upon recognition, and thus Donne can compare the manifestation of symptoms to the religious rite of confession: they are alike in that both function as a language (at one point he even refers to these physical spots as divine "hieroglyphs") that "declares" the nature of the disorder (86–88).

The various treatments that Donne undergoes, like the illness itself, are throughout interpreted as symbolic of spiritual realities: therapies for the body parallel therapies for the soul. As we have noted, one such treatment is placing pigeons at the feet of the ill person in order to "draw the vapours from the head." Donne understands this natural remedy for an illness of the body as analogous to divine remedies for ills of the soul as recorded in scripture: the laying of pigeons at the feet becomes a figure for the descent of the Holy Ghost in the form of a dove when Christ is baptized: "Therefore hast thou been pleased to afford us this remedy in nature, by this application of a dove to our lower parts, to make these vapours in our bodies to descend, and to make that a type to us, that, by the visitation of thy Spirit, the vapours of sin shall descend, and we tread them under our feet" (82). By the same logic of symbols, Donne compares purgation, the most common seventeenth-century treatment for illness, to the act of confession, for both involve a discharge of noxious substance: "peccant humours" are drawn out of the body in catharsis, and sins are purged from the soul in confession (135–36).

This analogy between sickness and sin is functional as well as interpretive: illness is purposive, sent by God both as punishment and as correction of sin. Disease not only reminds us of sin but exists so that we will do something about the state of our souls: repent, turn away from sin, and reform our lives. Over and over Donne assures himself that his sickness is intended as an occasion for repentance: "These corrections," he writes, "are the elements of our regeneration" (49). Illness for Donne is thus "not merely a natural accident" (41). It has a spiritual cause: "sin is the root and the fuel of all sickness"; it has a spiritual purpose: "this sickness is thy immediate correction"; and it has a spiritual function: "my sickness [is] an occasion of thy sending health" (48, 41, 26).

The analogy between sin and repentance, on the one hand, and illness and recovery, on the other, is central to attitudes about illness in Donne's time. And though Donne's recovery in the *Devotions* is not overtly associated with feelings of renewal and regeneration, the turning point in his illness conforms, structurally, to the archetype of conversion as it appears in religious autobiography. This is not surprising, especially when we reflect upon the fact that an illness, according to the Galenic medical model of Donne's time, was expected to develop or "ripen" until it reached its "crisis," at which point the patient, if he or she survived this, could expect to recover. The similarity between the older medical paradigm of illness, crisis, and recovery and the arc of the conversion archetype—which begins with the life of sin before conversion, reaches a climax in a conversion, and then concludes with the convert's reformed life afterwards—contributes to the coherence of Donne's religious formulation in the *Devotions.*

As we have observed, the progress of the illness in the *Devotions* is represented both as analogous to and as dependent upon the progress of the soul in understanding the meaning and right use of bodily illness. Thus the turning point in Donne's sickness is related not to any bodily change, nor to any therapeutic agent or procedure, but to a significant event in his spiritual life. Midway through the narrative, his thoughts, stimulated by the continuous tolling of bells for those who are dying, turn to the illness and death of others—and therewith to his own impending death. The psychological movement in these chapters is very subtle but absolutely central—and worth analyzing carefully.

These meditations begin with thoughts of a plurality of anonymous deaths, "the funerals of others," then move to focus on a single if impersonal and representative death, "he, for whose funeral these bells ring now," and then cluster around a more affective image, "this dead brother of ours" (105–6). In the next and most famous meditation, Donne turns from the dying man to himself—and to the reader, as well: "Any man's death diminishes me, because I am involved in mankind, and therefore never send to know for whom the bell tolls; it tolls for thee" (109). What Donne comes to realize is not simply that he, in his illness, is like a certain dying man, nor only that all mankind is subject to illness and death, but that we are all a part of a larger whole: "No man is an island, entire of itself; every man is a piece of the continent, a part of the main" (108). As he prays for the soul of his predecessor in death, he is praying for himself. And this is explicitly considered an act of *caritas* in the highest sense, where self and other become merged in the love of God. It is no accident that these chapters occur just after the appearance of the symptomatic spots and directly precede the first signs of Donne's recovery.

And what of the mortal instrument of Donne's recovery? The doctor in Donne's time is a figure with a good deal less power and importance than today. Twentieth-century pathographers, as we have seen, sometimes so value the abilities of their physicians that they tend to exaggerate them, but Donne feels the need to justify using a physician at all. He does so in accordance with the incarnational premises of Christianity, seeing the physician as God's agent on earth: "I know thou hast made the matter, and the man, and the art; and I go not from thee when I go to the physician" (25). However, he appends qualifiers to this "liberal" assertion. The doctor must be a practicing Christian if his therapies are to be at all helpful, and the patient must be cautious in his expectations of what his doctor can do. The sick person, Donne writes, is in error if he "casts himself wholly, entirely upon the physician, confides in him, relies upon him, attends all from him, and neglects that spiritual physic . . . instituted in thy Church" (26). The implicit therapeutic contract is one in which the patient agrees to be moderate in his expectations of what his physician can do for him, and the physician adopts a stance of humility in acknowledging that his medical skill—both the art and the science—comes from God.[12]

Most modern pathographies—popular books written by ordinary people—inevitably suffer in comparison to the *Devotions*, a work by a major poet and a theologian of formidable intellectual powers. Donne's pathography succeeds because the religious and the medical are consistently and masterfully interwoven: illness, in that it expresses the will of God, is determined to be meaningful; and medical treatment, interpreted as analogous to spiritual therapies, is given a higher purpose, whereas the physician is reduced to a position commensurate with his limited human abilities.[13] In contemporary pathographies with a religious frame of reference, however, this interconnection between two wholly different intellectual systems seems to have broken down. The result is an assortment of narratives where the formulation never quite succeeds in carrying the experience.

Donne's *Devotions* is characterized by a consistent and principled acceptance of either outcome of his illness—whether death or life. In contrast, most contemporary religious pathographies focus narrowly on the issue of cure, bypassing any attempt to find religious meaning in illness, in its treatment, and in the possibility of death.

There is, for example, Shireen Perry's *In Sickness and in Health*, a pathography about her 29-year-old husband's illness and death from AIDS. Both the Perrys are born-again Christians. Before his conversion, Mark Perry engaged in a gay life-style involving promiscuity and extensive drug use; with his conversion, he renounced homosexuality and gave up drugs, marrying three years later. When he discovers he has AIDS—only months after his marriage—he responds with the absolute and unshakable conviction that he will be healed by divine intervention. Though Perry does try both orthodox and alternative treatments, in the pathographical formulation (and, most probably, in the experience itself), therapies of any sort seem relatively unimportant. Religion is central to this pathography, and religious belief here seems to be reduced to the power of God to heal.

Accordingly, at one point Perry makes a formal confession of his previous homosexual life-style to a gathering of some two hundred church members, convinced that this has to be done before healing can occur. When he finds he is no better, he schedules another formal appearance before the church congregation; but again, the anticipated healing episode does not take place. At this point his mental condition deteriorates to the extent that he not only undergoes a crisis of faith but also begins acting strangely and displaying marked hostility and even paranoia toward family and friends.

One must wonder about the responses of Perry's wife—the author of the pathography—to all this: throughout, she depicts herself as a passive and helpless observer, a consistently selfless and loving wife. This uninflected authorial stance may account in part for the book's lack of psychological depth: it is possible that the author is defensively unreflective about the possible implications of her husband's experience.[14] When the book ends, Perry has overcome his anger and feelings of betrayal and dies surrounded by the love and support of his wife and church congregation. Despite this "happy" ending, the pathography cannot be said to have succeeded in achieving a religious formulation that renders the illness experience coherent and meaningful.

Terry Jones's *Venom in My Veins* is also a pathography written by a believing Christian. Like Perry's, this pathography focuses on cure. As Jones looks back over his life, he mentions early symptoms that proved difficult to diagnose, then a conversion-like experience that was followed by a message from God—"Healing through giving" (46). Soon afterwards a benefactor enables him to travel to the Mayo clinic for a medical workup, where he is told that he has amyotrophic lateral sclerosis (Lou Gehrig's disease), that nothing can be done, and that he may not have much time left. He then finds the same benefactor willing to pay his expenses for an experimental treatment program in Florida involving injections of cobra venom. When the progress of the disease appears to be halted by this treatment, he feels God calls him to become a full-time, traveling evangelist, convinced that this is what "healing through giving" really means. And he does become an evangelist, despite the severe physical handicaps that are a result of his illness—for example, he is unable to dress himself or even comb his hair.

Though Jones describes an enabling formulation, the pathography lacks the integration of medical and religious spheres that we found in Donne's

Devotions. What, for example, is the relationship between God and Jones's secular benefactor? And why cobra venom? The association of the serpent with sin or Satan goes back to the Garden of Eden. But Terry Jones, pastor of the Church of the Nazarene at the time he writes his pathography, never alludes to this association. It is unlikely that Donne's elaborate allegorical figures or metaphorical "conceits" would appear in any modern pathography. In a modern *religious* pathography, however, one might expect to find an attempt to organize medical phenomena in relation to some religious meaning. However, throughout Jones's pathography, as in Perry's, the medical and the secular are not so much interpreted through a religious frame of reference as drastically subordinated to it or divorced from it. Nowhere do we sense any real attempt at understanding the spiritual meaning of either illness or treatment.

A third religious pathography is the Rev. Clifford Oden's *Thank God I Have Cancer!*—a shrill and dogmatic defense of the use of Laetrile in treating the author's cancer of the colon. Unlike Perry and Jones, this author, a Baptist minister, eschews orthodox medicine altogether, seeing all authorities and institutions—religious and medical and political alike—as intrinsically evil because they represent "the world," and Satan is the prince of this world. More specifically, he believes that Satan is strongly involved in the anti-Laetrile campaign. Oden is convinced that just as God created the malignant cancer cell, so also He created a substance in nature to control it: "vitamin B-17," amygdalin. Healing is thus necessarily a "natural" process. Oden reduces the traditional association between sin and disease to bad living habits. If we live right—which means clean air, good food, and proper exercise—then we will not get sick. His attitude toward physicians is dogmatically skeptical: "God heals, your body heals, but doctors do not heal" (31). The physician "can facilitate healing" but only if he or she cooperates with "God's principles of healing," which Oden insists are rooted in the essential goodness of nature. Since amygdalin is a substance derived from apricot pits and thus "natural," and since amygdalin is a source of Laetrile, then this is the therapy intended by God for cancer treatment. This pathography succeeds in achieving a formulation that does, in a sense, bring together the spheres of medicine and religion—but it does so only by absorbing the whole of medicine into a worldview that seems less Christian than Manichaean and perhaps even paranoid.

Each of these three pathographies is limited in the way it uses religious constructs to understand and deal with illness. At first glance James L.

Johnson's *Coming Back*, discussed earlier in this chapter, seems to inter-weave religious and medical constructs more successfully. Johnson's path-ography differs from all other religious pathographies, including Donne's, in that he appears to have undergone some sort of mystical experience as a direct result of his medical condition. Johnson refers to two visions, one of Heaven and one of Hell, that occur just after his bypass surgery. His description of these visions is tantalizingly allusive: "I knew I had seen something, been beyond myself, outside myself, in other dimensions," he writes at one point; and elsewhere he refers to "those dimensions I had been in, those 'outside' territories beyond life" but adds that "I didn't know, or will never know, how to explain them" (93, 95). The experience, even though he cannot explain it, undoubtedly has an impact on the changes in values and life-style that result from his heart attack: though admitting that he has had "no great heavenly vision as such," he feels that he has been given "a whole new consciousness of the immensity of God against the small-fry dimensions of man" (98).

Despite the fact that one acknowledges the genuineness of Johnson's experience, at the same time one is left with little more than his repeated allusions to it. All his vision seems to produce is the recognition of the need to slow down so typical of the pathographies of many heart attack patients, religious or not. Johnson's pathography really does not achieve a formula-tion in which the medical and the religious interface. For example, though references to God are frequent, there is little evidence here of the kind of spiritual soul-searching characteristic of Donne's *Devotions*, nor of the psychological self-analysis so often found in secular pathographies. As Johnson himself explicitly states in his prologue, his condition of "spiritual heart disease . . . has nothing to do with sin or not being a Christian." What it does reflect is a "spiritual workaholic life" of stress and frantic ac-tivity. The examination of conscience in this book goes no further than the superficialities of living too fast and too hard: it does not probe the depths of psyche or soul. In some sense, then, this book offers formula rather than formulation.

Of all those I have read, Lois Walfred Johnson's pathography seems among the most successful in bringing together the beliefs and practices of Christianity and the language and concepts of scientific medicine. Lois Johnson's story begins when she discovers a lump in her breast: the lump is biopsied, found to be malignant, and treated by mastectomy and che-motherapy. Eighteen months later another lump is discovered, which

proves benign. But she tells us little of her experience with doctors, therapies, hospitals, or even her illness itself: like other religious pathographies,
her narrative is characterized by a single-minded focus on the religious
aspects of her experience.

The title of the pathography is itself a précis of the author's stance and
the book's content and focus: *Either Way, I Win: A Guide for Growth in the
Power of Prayer*. Prayer is seen and used as a potent therapeutic tool, a spiritual aid to conventional medical therapies: "Praying effectively involves my
diagnosing harmful germs," explains Johnson, "asking Christ to immunize
me against them" (82). Prayer and religious healing are for her therapies
that complement orthodox medicine; they are not intended to replace it.
Thus she argues that "those refusing to use doctors or medicine limit God"
(172–73). Throughout the book the spiritual and the physical are treated
as parallel dimensions. Over and over she refers to her cancer as "physical
cancer" (9, 27)—as opposed to emotional or spiritual cancer: "There are
many forms of cancer. It's natural to think first of the kind seen under a
microscope, yet there are also cancers of fear, hurt, depression, loneliness
and unbelief" (9). Medicine, for her, is only one form of knowledge—thus
she frequently begins a sentence with "Medically, I know . . ." Similarly,
medical therapies are perceived as only one kind of treatment for one kind
of disease.

In her views on healing, Lois Johnson diverges from the narrow concern with bodily cure characteristic of the three other religious pathographies—Shireen Perry's, Terry Jones's, and Rev. Clifford Oden's. She is
herself a healer who works by laying on of hands, though she does not seem
to see a parallel between herself and her physicians, or perhaps she chooses
not to comment on it. Healing itself is something that can occur on several levels—the physical, the emotional, or the spiritual: "every person who
asks receives some form of healing" (169). The fact that some of these
people do not get well indicates not failure but only that God has chosen
some other kind of healing for them. She remarks, moreover, that death is
not an indication that healing has not occurred, since the death of the body
is a kind of ultimate healing for the Christian (172).

At first glance the attitudes in this pathography seem similar to those
of Donne's *Devotions*. Both share a pervasive dualism of physical and spiritual realities, though the habit of dualism in Lois Johnson's pathography
is a fuzzy one, lacking the precise isomorphic relationships between physical and spiritual therapies—purgation and confession, for example—so

striking in Donne's pathography. For both authors the importance of the illness, of physicians and therapies, and of the possibility of death is diminished; instead, precedence is given to spiritual realities.

Johnson's pathography, however, departs from its older counterpart in her attitude toward the relation of sin and illness. For Donne, as we have seen, illness is perceived as a sign of some underlying spiritual disorder. Johnson's attitude is more like that of modern pathographers in that she pointedly rejects the association of cancer with "a dreadful sin" (156). She does ask if her illness might signify some kind of spiritual disorder, and she does suggest that sick people should go through the exercise of "search[ing] their hearts"; but the language in which she couches her own self-questioning suggests the shallowness of her search: "Is there something in my life needing correction? Have I done something foolish, bringing this upon myself? Working without enough rest, for instance?" (54–55). Most of us, if we are honest with ourselves, could easily find evidence of far more serious sins than "working without rest."

The difference here between Johnson and Donne, the twentieth-century and the seventeenth-century believer, is considerable: Donne uses his illness as an occasion for self-diagnosis and, presumably finding evidence of spiritual pathology, uses his attempts to recover from illness as the occasion for spiritual growth. Johnson, on the contrary, seems to turn away both from her illness and from any sense of sin in her focus on the religious life. But it is precisely an author's concern with the interior condition of psyche or spirit that gives personal narrative of all kinds its depth. In this, pathographies organized explicitly around a religious frame of reference seem unsuccessful, not only in comparison to Donne's *Devotions* but also when contrasted with contemporary secular pathographies.

Though our sample is too small to allow generalizations that are reliable or fair, one cannot help registering a sense of disappointment in pathographies written out of some form of religious orthodoxy. They seem thin, especially when compared to a work like Donne's *Devotions*. In part this is due simply to the vast cultural shifts between his time and our own, the change from a world of analogies and symbols to a world of facts. For Jones, there is no significance in the snake venom that he swallows as if it were any other remedy, but for Donne any serpent is the serpent in the Garden, whose venom is sin.[15] And for Schwerin—though we do not know if she is Christian—it is improbable that the real pigeons resting and feeding outside her windows would serve, like the pigeons laid at Donne's feet, as figures for the Holy Spirit.

Yet the thinness we sense in modern religious pathographies cannot be explained entirely by the sense that we live in a secular and scientific age. Paradoxically, it may be precisely because the authors *are so* often born-again Christians that their pathographies fail to explore fully the potential for religious meaning in their sickness and recovery (or death). The problem is one of synchronization: these authors are already converted before they ever fall sick, and therefore their illness cannot be the occasion for their change of heart. The point becomes especially clear in Perry's pathography, where conversion and illness are linked, if not synchronous. Since Mark Perry's illness presumably results from sexual practices he renounces as sinful at the time of his conversion, the appearance of AIDS either threatens the validity and meaning of his conversion or else calls into question God's justice. The public confessions he arranges can be interpreted as his attempt to salvage both: Perry sets the stage for God to perform a miraculous healing that would verify the conversion and validate His redemptive powers. Everything, then, turns on cure.

But Donne, too, was converted before he fell ill. Dr. Donne, Dean of Saint Paul's, is no longer Jack Donne, the libertine poet of the "Songs and Sonnets": he has put away his former self in a conversion that makes him— in the eyes of his biographer, Izaak Walton—a second Augustine.[16] However, as Donne realizes (and Perry may not), conversion is an ongoing process as well as an event, and the work of repentance ends only with life itself: "I have had three births," Donne writes in his dedication to the *Devotions*, "one, natural, when I came into the world; one, supernatural, when I entered into the ministry; and now, a preternatural birth, in returning to life, from this sickness" (3). The difference in the way the two men— Donne and Perry—interpret the link that both accept between sin and illness is striking; and it accounts in part for the fact that for Donne the myth is enabling, but for Perry, disastrous—misunderstood and misapplied.

In one way, then, Donne's *Devotions* may be closer to the contemporary secular pathography than to the religious pathographies we have considered, for it deals with conversion in mythic rather than literal terms. And this helps us see that the attitudes toward sickness so powerfully depicted in the *Devotions* have not vanished nor have they been replaced by a purely medicoscientific understanding of illness. What seems to have happened is that the *"ars morbi"* that was so much a part of a specifically Christian frame of reference in the seventeenth century has, in our time, become subsumed and disseminated into a culture that is largely secular. The essential myth, then, persists. The sense that recovery from a serious illness is like a rebirth, the feeling that illness can be an occasion for spiritual growth, the association between illness and sin—though these attitudes often seem strangely absent from religious pathographies, they are present, as we have seen (and will see, in chapter 5) in a wide variety of pathographies that acknowledge no explicit religious referent.

✛

CHAPTER THREE

Myths of Battle and Journey

Metaphors of battle and journey are ubiquitous in pathography. Indeed, the pervasiveness of these metaphors suggests that they have become an inherent part of our way of experiencing ourselves and the world. Both motifs have their roots in the deepest strata of our culture: Homer's *Iliad* is an epic of heroic warfare and his *Odyssey* an epic of heroic quest; the more ancient *Gilgamesh* combines both. It is likely that metaphors of battle and quest predate these texts, since they are readily found in the myths and legends of a great variety of cultures, where they frequently occur in tandem.[1] In pathography, journey and battle become very different mythic paradigms with different associations, implications, and associated images. Each must be examined in turn.

The Battle Myth

There are really two paradigms for the battle motif in ancient literature and myth: the battle between human hero and monstrous foe and the cosmic warfare between different kinds of divinities.[2] The two paradigms are alike in that the gods represent perfected images of the human, whereas their adversaries tend to be giants, monsters, or hybrids of the animal and the human. So in Greek mythology, Zeus must overthrow the child-devouring Kronos and his Titans as well as defeat the giants, hundred-handed monsters like Briareus and Enceladus or fire-breathing creatures like Typhon. In the Christian tradition, Lucifer and his dark angels rebel against God, only to be defeated and cast down by Saint Michael and the heavenly host. In Norse mythology, Odin slays the giant Ymir and forms the world out of his body; he must then chain the wolf Fenris, cast out the Midgard serpent and Hela, who is death, and eventually bind Loki, the father of all three monsters. A striking feature of all these myths is that the adversaries of the gods are not destroyed like the foes of human heroes but are bound and restrained: the Titans are imprisoned in Tartaros and the giants under Aetna; Satan and his devils are thrown down to hell, also deep within the earth; Ymir is buried at the root of Yggdrasill, the world tree; and Loki and his children are cast out or put in bondage—temporarily. For in both Christian and Norse myth, there is (to modify the Freudian phrase) a 'return of the suppressed': the battle at the beginning will recur at the end, when Michael will again face Satan, and Odin and his heroes will confront Loki and his allies. The gods, it seems, fight at the beginning and the end, while human heroes carry on what is essentially the same battle in between.

At the deepest level, both these paradigms of battle—the human and the divine—concern the ancient idea of the world as organized around (or out of) the struggle between light and darkness, life and death, good and evil. The "mythogenic" habit in Western culture of thinking in oppositions and in contrarieties has influenced the way we think about other things as well: health and disease, for example. Health seems to fit in naturally with those entities that protect and nurture humanity—light, life, and good; disease, correspondingly, belongs with darkness, death, and evil. As I hope to show, a good many of the mythic components in our attitudes about health and illness derive from this sort of agonistic thinking—from a conception of the world as composed of matched sets of antagonistic principles.

This dualistic, antagonistic model is one that has been reinforced, over and over, in Western culture.[3] Though Christianity in its most orthodox form appears at first glance to be monistic—God is the only reality, evil is but the perversion or privation of good, Hell is the place where God's justice is enacted, and Satan is really in God's employ, his powers to tempt and to torture being in a sense "on loan"—a powerful philosophic dualism is and always has been deeply embedded in the Christian mythos. Thus the Epistles of Paul draw a stark opposition between flesh and spirit, implying that all flesh is evil and all that is spirit is good. Augustine was himself at one time a believer in the duality of good and evil; and though this belief was condemned as the Manichaean heresy and its proponents persecuted, it has survived throughout the history of Christianity to emerge at various intervals, only to be condemned again as heretical. Medieval Christianity is permeated by a kind of latent Manichaeism in its opposition of the Trinity of Father, Son, and Holy Spirit to the evil triad of the World, the Flesh, and the Devil; in the opposition of the seven Virtues, Christian and cardinal, to the seven Deadly Sins; and in the metaphor familiar to us from the morality play of the believer as a kind of battlefield where the forces of good and evil, God and Satan, fight for possession of the soul. With Protestantism, this dualism is only intensified: for the Elect, Calvin observes, repentance is "a warfare [to] be terminated only by death" (*Institutes,* III.ii.ix, 658).

Christianity's habit of dualism becomes an explicit military metaphor in the familiar passage from Ephesians urging the believer to "put on the whole armor of God" and with the breastplate of righteousness, the shield of faith, the helmet of salvation, and the sword of the spirit, to fight against the "rulers of the darkness of this world" (6: 11–17). The metaphor becomes historical reality in the Crusades: the Christian crusader believed that he fought for God and truth and goodness against the Infidel, who represented falsehood and evil. For centuries afterward, the image of the faithful Christian knight battling the armies of sin and Satan remained a central metaphor for the way the Christian was to behave on earth. This image of the knight was again literalized in World War I, with the British soldier depicted in war posters as a knight in shining armor—often surrounded by angels or accompanied by some divine sign of his messianic calling—fighting against that twentieth-century infidel, "the Hun" (Girouard).

Given this history of the image of the knight battling Evil, it seems appropriate that many cancer patients who try to strengthen the body's immune system by guided mental imagery picture a knight or an army of knights on horseback defeating subhuman beings; the knights represent white blood cells or chemical agents, and the subhuman beings stand for the cancer cells (Simonton 1980, 153, fig. 3; Achterberg, figs. 22, 24, and 25). In fact (according to Achterberg and Lawlis), the most common symbol of the immune system in cancer patients' visualizations is the white knight: "The symbols of positive connotation are those representing strength and purity; powerful enough to subdue an enemy—pure enough to do so with justification. Such images frequently take the form of knights" (94).

The pervasiveness of military metaphor in our contemporary understanding of illness and its therapies is thus not at all surprising; indeed it seems almost predetermined. We often understand disease as the consequence of a breach in the body's "defense-system," a concept that seems very much a function of our habit of thinking militarily: microorganisms invade the body and try to take over while white blood cells quickly come to the body's defense and attack the alien entities; if they conquer them, health is restored. Treatment is similarly militaristic. Common therapies include antibiotics to combat infectious diseases of all sorts, radiation to eradicate enemy cancer cells, and a vast arsenal of chemical weapons— some proven effective, some still experimental—employed in the attempt to cure or retard a disease such as cancer or AIDS or to control illnesses such as diabetes or lupus or heart disease.[4]

At this point, the relevance of the hero battling monsters or the cosmic battle between divine and diabolic forces becomes obvious. In a real sense, the world of medicine in the West mirrors the world of myth: our therapies are the weapons by which we battle the exogenous monsters of disease entities like cancer or AIDS, and what we call cure is most often a remission in which these "beasts" are suppressed, controlled, chained beneath the surface of our "healthy" lives. For every cure, however complete, and every remission, however long, is only temporary. Eventually, for each one of us, some terminal disease or ultimate system failure will triumph, and death will result. In this, medical fact again resonates with mythic paradigm: the fact that our own personal lives will come to an end finds a macrocosmic equivalent in the myth of the Christian Armageddon or the Norse Ragnarok—that final battle between the divine and the demonic or bestial that will destroy the world and life as we know it.

The habit of associating military metaphors with disease and therapy is one that is reinforced by social and political factors. One is the typically American blending of an aggressive stance with an almost naive social optimism, evidenced in recent political slogans appropriated from the military sphere as the "war on poverty" or the "war on cancer," or, more recently, the "war on drugs." The ideology behind these pseudomilitary campaigns suggests that poverty or cancer or drugs are not endemic to society but antisocial foes that can be conquered, if only we fight hard enough. Lyndon Johnson is responsible for the "war on poverty," a phrase coined in the early part of his administration; and Richard Nixon, in imitation of Johnson, introduced the "war on cancer" not long thereafter (Bailey). It may be of interest that both slogans emerged well after World War II in a period marked by the unpopular Vietnam war, by the ubiquitous presence of the Cold War, and by threats of an imminent nuclear war. Perhaps these slogans can be seen both as sublimating and displacing martial energies not satisfied in the ambiguous "wars" of the time; perhaps, too, they can be seen as deflecting a possible World War III. Aggressive energies felt as terrifying in the context of nuclear war are here defused and made useful by directing them onto such enemies as cancer or poverty.

Our association between the military and the medical is also reinforced by the way scientific medicine tends to reify certain medical conditions as disease entities and then see these disease entities as separate from the life and body of the patient. Our epistemologies of disease do influence the way we treat it. Disease is most commonly perceived as exogenous, as alien, as lacking any organic relation to the person who is ill: thus certain illnesses, especially cancer, are characterized by treatment modalities aimed primarily at attacking the disease, not treating the individual whose body is affected by the disease.[5] This is the model we have successfully used against infectious diseases, and it seems hard for us to see it as a model with very real limitations. But it is not only doctors who prefer the exogenous model; patients, too, instinctively think in this way. Thus a popular understanding of minor illnesses would divide them into bacterial or viral infections; both are introduced from outside in the form of microorganisms. One often hopes an infection is bacterial, because then antibiotics will be prescribed and these will "knock out" the invading germs.

Yet another factor contributing to the association between military metaphor and illness—or perhaps one deriving from it—is the recent discovery, popularized by media channels and legitimized in the claim that it is "scientific," that passive, compliant patients fare less well in surviving a serious illness than their aggressive and noncompliant counterparts. Kenneth Shapiro declares in his pathography: "It is a well-documented fact that those people who have the mental tenacity to fight do better than those who just quit" (9). Similarly, Joyce Slayton Mitchell, in *Winning the Chemo Battle,* alludes to "scientific evidence" that demonstrates "that cancer patients who have a fighting spirit and who don't accept a negative verdict are far more likely to improve than those who stoically accept feelings of helplessness and hopelessness" (203). A stance such as this, often legitimized by referring to scientific statistics and studies, is pervasive in pathography, as patients with various illnesses concentrate their energies on "fighting" their disease, or the effect of their therapies, or their own attitude. The "battle" must be waged on all fronts.

In view of the overwhelming cultural predisposition toward making use of the battle myth and of the way it is reinforced in America today, we must ask whether it is one that proves helpful or unhelpful in actual situations of illness.[6] Here pathography is eminently useful, because it can show us how a given myth functions in particular cases. The idea that illness is a battle between a disease and its therapeutic agents occurs over and over in pathographies of all kinds. In many cases it serves to enhance the ill person's sense of dignity, self-esteem, and active participation in therapy. In other instances, though, the myth functions in such a way that the sick person becomes the battlefield, or the energies of both doctor and patient are displaced onto fighting the disease rather than helping the human being who is sick.

The military myth seems particularly appropriate to cancer, since cancer is so often characterized as an alien intruder or an invading enemy, and its various therapies considered as weapons with which to attack or destroy the disease. As we might expect, military imagery is found in a great many pathographies about cancer. The protagonist in one pathography, hospitalized for terminal leukemia, sums up this attitude: "It's like going to war," he writes, "only the battlefield is inside my body. I have to fight a battle with the enemy and destroy it. This damn disease is my enemy—it is trying to kill me" (Panger, 160). Similarly, a woman with ovarian cancer observes (in a chapter entitled "The War"): "Now here I was, deeply embroiled in the battle of my life—a war against cancer taking place in my own body" (Radner, 124); Deena Metzger describes her mastectomy for breast cancer as "sacrificing a battalion to save the war" (165), and Audre Lorde repeatedly characterizes herself, post-mastectomy, as an "Amazon warrior." As these examples demonstrate, military imagery seems readily accessible to ill persons as they describe their experiences. Significantly, too, it is a metaphoric construct often shared by the doctors who treat them. Thus a lymphoma patient quotes a hospital psychiatrist as urging him: "You must treat every malignant cell as an enemy, then fight it to the limit" (Widome, 137). And a young woman with cancer of the thyroid expresses her surprise at the way her physician explains her therapy in "nuclear terms, using the words 'bombardment' and 'destruction,'" and then goes on to adopt this kind of metaphor in her own attitude toward her illness: "I felt ready to fight and to make any sacrifice to vanquish the disease" (Paoli, 56, 99).

It is unfortunate that for one pathographer, the war against the disease at times becomes a war against the research oncologists she consults. Barbara Creaturo is a forty-three-year-old woman who aggressively studies various promising experimental treatments for ovarian cancer, the research oncologists associated with them, and the hospitals or research clinics where such programs are available—and who feels she has thereby acquired a reputation as a "difficult patient." At one point, as she deliberates how to find out about a promising experimental protocol without risking the ire of her present oncologist, she writes: "I'm weary of fighting this unwinnable war against a phalanx of doctors, all armored in their invincible authority. Why must I be so frightened, not just of my disease but of the doctors who are supposed to be helping me defeat it?" (168–69).

In part, the popularity and usefulness of the metaphor of battle may be related to the strong aversion felt by many ill people, especially women, to the idea of themselves as victims. So Jory Graham, in a pathography that seems primarily concerned with the negative image of cancer and cancer patients, deplores the popular association of cancer with what is dirty and foul, and sees the term "cancer victim" as an "odious label." Too often, in literature and in real life, women are cast in the role of victim: in revolt against this, the metaphor of fighting an illness connotes strength and masculinity. For some patients, it also suggests control: Mitchell observes in her pathography that "as soon as we begin to fight, we take control; we change the quality of our life" (203).

Cornelius and Kathryn Ryan's *A Private Battle* turns this kind of occasional imagery of warfare into a sustained allegorical figure. The fact that Ryan, a military historian, writes the story of his cancer experience at the same time as his final book about World War II, *A Bridge Too Far,* makes it clear that his comparison of the world of illness and the world of war is a conscious one. The likeness between illness and war for Ryan is both descriptive and functional; not only does he see an analogy between his private battle with cancer and the historical battle, but he is able to exploit those analogies to help him live with cancer and die from it with the courage and dignity that he so values.

A Private Battle is permeated with references to war. Ryan's cancer is of course the enemy, the therapies function as weapons, his many helpful friends recall the courageous civilians of the Resistance, and his physicians are like the various generals of World War II about whom he writes in his histories. The initial surgical procedure is referred to as an attack, the possibility of further metastases as a "counterattack," and his physician's later recourse to estrogen therapy as a "second line of defense" against "the enemy." Remission means a temporary success for the forces of treatment; relapse a victory for the foe. Ryan himself in this private allegory becomes a commander-in-chief, who, in consultation with his generals, plans the military strategy that best promises success. And in the end, Ryan sees himself as a brave and courageous soldier who dies fighting—who does not ever really "give up."

The change from seeing himself as commander-in-chief to seeing himself as an ordinary soldier demonstrates how Ryan makes the analogy with war into an enabling myth, for each role embodies what he needs at specific stages in the development of his illness. The image of commander-in-chief suggests an aggressive, decisive stance; that of soldier suggests a more passive, less controlling image. The success of the military myth, for Ryan, results from his ability to adapt it to his needs—needs that change during the course of the illness. After all the many battles fought in the long campaign between those two enemies—cancer and its treatments—the war finally ends with the triumph of the disease. But at the same time, the value he places on winning the battle undergoes a transformation in which survival becomes subordinate to something else. For when Ryan learns that his efforts to reverse his illness have not succeeded, he transposes the entire war to another level, where what matters is not winning or losing but such qualities as courage, compassion, pride, and heroism.

But the military myth that here serves Ryan as an enabling device can also be disabling. Martha Weinman Lear's *Heartsounds* is an account of her husband's struggles with and eventual death from atherosclerotic heart disease. Harold Lear is a physician in his fifties who suffers a massive myocardial infarction. He undergoes open-heart surgery that, though successful, results in an undetermined degree of brain damage—a result initially denied by his physicians. *Heartsounds* documents Lear's "fight" against heart disease—his attempt to continue the same "battle" that he was involved in as a physician, but this time from the other side, as a patient. Thus Martha Lear describes a postsurgical nightmare where her husband calls out repeatedly, *"Where is my adversary?"* She observes: "It was the neat surgical mind demanding an adversary, an enemy, a pathology, recognizable forces of death and disease against which he might pit his own skills." She goes on to remark that his medical training had conditioned him to regard illness as "a *thing*"—a germ, a kidney-stone, a cancer, an infection —and to view his own role as physician as one in which he actively fights the disease, not passively and helplessly endures it (151–52).

The tone of this book combines confusion and deepening despair on the part of Lear with rage and helplessness on the part of his wife.

Heartsounds is a virtual encyclopedia of all the horrors of which institutional medicine is capable: callousness from the house staff, arrogance and evasiveness from the specialists involved, and numerous errors in medical procedures—both major and minor. Thus, on one occasion, Lear nearly dies when an intern refuses to respond to his call for medical attention; at another time, the lining of his stomach is damaged when huge doses of potassium are administered without liquids; later still, he is given anesthesia for a coronary angiography after the procedure is virtually completed.

Despite the fact that both Ryan and Lear eventually die from their illnesses, the difference in tone, attitude, and outlook between these two pathographies is striking. Both men are comfortable with military metaphors and models—Lear in his role as physician and Ryan through his books on war. The personalities of both men seem aggressive, forceful, controlling. For Ryan, the military myth seems to work to his advantage because he is able to adapt it to personal needs that change as the illness progresses. For Lear, though, this does not happen; the military metaphor never works very well at all as an enabling myth, and he is unable either to disregard it or to replace it with something else.[7]

It would seem that the military myth, in order to function in an enabling way, requires certain conditions surrounding the illness: there must be an adversary, an enemy "other," something that can be identified, measured, and then combatted; the patient must feel that the physicians are allies in the battle against disease; and there must be some therapeutic agent or procedure that can act as weaponry. None of these conditions exists in the Lear narrative. Thus the military myth fails here not because Lear dies (for this is also true of Ryan) but because of the ambiguous nature of his medical problem and because his own experience of his condition is at variance with the judgment of his physicians. The result of a situation where the military myth is operative without an appropriate "enemy" and without medical "allies" in the battle against disease is manifested in the angry tone that predominates throughout the Lear pathography. The energies aroused by this myth, lacking any appropriate inimical forces, are displaced onto the potential "allies," the patient's physicians, or simply left without an object and released as a measureless rage or a profound bitterness. It is also true that Lear's primary medical problem is cardiac disease, whereas Ryan's is cancer. Perhaps the battle metaphor is more often enabling when it is associated with a disease involving the body's immunological system, since that conforms to contemporary medicine's elaborately military explanations of how the immunological system functions. The metaphor of fighting one's disease would appear to be most prevalent in pathographies about cancer, but this may simply reflect the fact that there are so many more pathographies written about cancer than about other diseases.

The military metaphor is also widespread in pathographies about AIDS.[8] Emmanuel Dreuilhe's *Mortal Embrace* uses the war metaphor so extensively that he himself describes it as an allegory (43). His autobiography is "a warrior's discourse," he refers to dealing with AIDS as "the war effort," AIDS itself is "a tank pulverizing everything in its path," and his therapies are "an artillery barrage of antiviral and sulfa drugs" that are "chemical weapons in the trench warfare." He refers to himself sometimes as a "war casualty" and sometimes as a "Resistance fighter" devoted "to throwing off the foreign viral yoke"; his doctors are military officers, hospitals are trenches or war zones whose admission rituals produce "a militarization of conduct" (7, 28, 7, 17, 77–78). AIDS, he remarks, is World War III, and AIDS patients are waiting for "another Oppenheimer [to] discover the fearsome weapon that will resolve this internal dissension and sweep the virus from the face of the earth" (18–19).

As this last quotation so eloquently demonstrates, *Mortal Embrace* seems to be written principally out of the author's feelings of rage and resentment. When we reflect, however, that Dreuilhe is not only trying to come to terms with his own disease but is also grieving for his lover, who recently died of AIDS, we can understand why the war metaphor seems here to reflect his anger more than any process of formulation. The allusions to war in this book are overwhelming, yet in the long run they seem superficial. The author finds evidence of his martial allegory everywhere, but he does not seem to *use* it, as other authors have, to help him better understand and deal with his situation.

This issue of the usefulness of a particular mythic paradigm is a very important one and requires further scrutiny. The metaphor of "fighting" disease is also pervasive in *The Screaming Room*, Barbara Peabody's pathography about her son's illness and death from AIDS. "AIDS is constant warfare," she observes, "an unending siege. The patient is like a small, weakly defended country surrounded by mighty powers. It fights fiercely to defend itself from invasion, but its weapons are few and primitively inadequate" (201).

Clearly, the battle myth is one that is helpful for Peabody, but several passages in this pathography cause one to wonder whether it is as helpful for her son, Peter. For example, she mentions Peter's tendency in dealing with challenges to give up too easily and too soon. She commends him in his battle against AIDS, but her commendation seems oddly qualified: "He's fighting. He hasn't given up, as I feared he might have, as he's done before" (18). Perhaps this man is at some deep level not someone for whom combat, struggle, and fighting are desirable ways of coping with illness. Recollections of the past and episodes from the present that Peabody includes in her book tend to confirm this possibility. Thinking back to his childhood, she mentions his refusal to engage in the rough-and-tumble play of young boys; now, she remarks on the way he tries to avoid suffering or violence on television. Indeed, an interview she describes between her son and an AIDS clinic social worker suggests that Peter does not find an aggressive stance helpful as a coping device. The social worker (whom he likes) tries to rouse his feelings of anger—at the disease, at his doctors, at anything. But Peter resolutely refuses to play along. His mother perceives him as exhausted and perhaps hurt by the interview, but she does not take the next step and conclude that admitting and expressing anger is not the way he would choose to deal with his situation.

In this pathography, then, the military myth seems helpful for the author, but much less so for her son, the person who is actually sick. The ambiguity about this myth is demonstrable in two consecutive statements —one about Peter and the other about the author herself. She remarks, "The fight will last as long as [Peter] wishes." But her very next sentence betrays whose fight this is: "I have come to realize what it really means to be a mother, to fight for your child" (27).

Perhaps it is possible, as Bernie Siegel has observed, that some people are "fighters" and some, simply, are not. In *Beyond AIDS*, George Melton is clear in defining his own stance as markedly different from that of the patient who is a "fighter." He remarks, "I knew my health would not come as a result of fighting my illness, but rather as a by-product of seeking my connection to the power within me" (35). Melton by temperament seems very much a pacifist. In explaining his decision to discontinue medication, he argues, "The virus was not really the enemy. There was no enemy without. . . . He who wields force is weak. Only in the laying down of all defense is true strength recognized" (68). Melton reports that for his lover, Wil, also stricken with ARC (AIDS Related Complex, a term now rarely used for symptoms that often lead to AIDS), military thinking is likewise unhelpful: finding himself uncomfortable with the military imagery so frequently encouraged in visualization exercises, Wil determines to imagine "love energy totally enveloping the virus" instead of "a war against the virus" (71–72).

A more complex and more ambiguous example of the use of military metaphor is Paul Monette's *Borrowed Time,* a masterfully written account of his lover's nineteen-month illness and eventual death from AIDS. The pathography is informed by the fact that Monette knows that he has AIDS himself. "I don't know if I will live to finish this" is the very first sentence of the book—a sober beginning. Military imagery is pervasive in this pathography and is central to the book's formulation. Throughout, AIDS is referred to as "The War," and everything—events, people, feelings—is perceived and understood in this context. As Anne Hudson Jones has observed, even the cover photograph is about war in its depiction of a Greek warrior holding his shield on one arm and supporting a fallen comrade with the other (10). Monette describes the onset of AIDS with powerful military imagery: "Suddenly you are at high noon in full battle gear. They have neglected to tell you that you will be issued no weapons of any sort. So you cobble together a weapon out of anything that lies at hand. . . . You fight tough, you fight dirty, but you cannot fight dirtier than it" (2). At this early stage, Monette naively assumes everything will be all right because "we would fight this thing like demons" (8). The warriors in this battle are himself and his lover, "the group of two for an army" (101)—an allusion to those heroic duos of Homeric epic, Achilleus and Patroklos or Sarpedon and Glaukos. This bellicose response to the disease seems almost reflexive and is seen as necessary in dealing with the depression that so easily accompanies an illness that is at this point in time both terrible and fatal.

In pathographies about AIDS (unlike many about cancer), it is primarily the patient, not the physician, who aggressively pursues experimental therapies and insists on treatment at all stages of the disease. The search for "the magic bullet" is a major theme in *Borrowed Time* and is seen as an intrinsic part of the battle against AIDS. So the author observes that "tracking down a cure . . . became a kind of compulsion, and gave me the best shot at a positive attitude" (99). Not infrequently, authors of pathographies will accuse their doctors of neglecting their patients' needs as persons in the scientific pursuit of a cure; here, the situation is dramatically reversed. The author, in concert with a network of others in the gay community, becomes an expert on immunology, learning how to discover and pursue the very latest experimental therapy and to acquire drugs still not legally permissible.

The military myth seems helpful to both the author and his lover primarily in fending off a despair that in this pathography seems always imminent. "Fighting was to despair," writes Monette, "what aspirin was to fever" (102–3). But besides alleviating their own psychological anguish, their efforts in the war on AIDS, he feels, contribute to a victory for later generations. Had a cure been found when the book was written, its author would surely have felt vindicated in his aggressive stance, and he probably would have felt this whether or not his friend, Roger, survived. Monette sees Roger as among the first to die in the long "battle against AIDS," a war where the fighters now are a "new generation" whose future looks brighter: "*Living with AIDS* is a rallying cry now, and the men of '85 were the first division to hum a few bars" (142).

In fact, though, no cure is found, and Roger is subjected to painful diagnostic and therapeutic medical procedures only to succumb to the disease in the end. In this context, the reverse aspect of the military myth becomes all too clear—for the emphasis in this book on an aggressive search for a cure is accompanied by an attitude of total denial toward death. When the diagnosis of AIDS is first made, the two men tell their doctor that they choose to see it "not as a death sentence but rather as a life challenge" (80). At a much later point, when a supportive and sympathetic nurse asks whether they had talked about how they would handle Roger's dying, Monette reports that "with some defiance" he answered, "No, we haven't. . . . We talk about fighting" (242). By this point the myth they share has become disabling: for both men, energy is focused on battling the disease and looking for a "magic cure" that never materializes, so that nothing is left over to deal with their feelings about Roger's impending death and Monette's future with AIDS. And Monette seems to recognize this problem. He refers to himself (at the time the incidents took place) as "living a total illusion" about Roger's chances for survival and, in retrospect, admits that he wishes they could have talked about their feelings (292). Given the degree of denial, which seems quite probably a function of the strength of the military myth, this proved impossible.

The war metaphor always seems to imply some degree of ambivalence, perhaps because it embodies both the glory of heroism and the horror of suffering and death. A paradigm that bears obvious resemblance to the military myth but avoids this ambivalence is the analogy between the patient and the athlete. Illness is here subsumed into the conventions of a sport, where how the game is played counts almost as much as who wins.

Moreover, this paradigm is reassuring in that athletics connotes health, the body tuned and developed to its finest possibility. And in this emphasis on physical fitness, there is an implicit antithesis and antidote to the debility of sickness. The fact that amyotrophic lateral sclerosis is more commonly known as "Lou Gehrig's disease" suggests that the athlete who is mortally ill may already belong to the dimension of the mythic.

Pathographies about athletes with a terminal illness are always marked by poignancy: we are moved by the plight of the young person in prime physical condition who nonetheless falls sick and soon after dies—an image with obvious resemblance to what happens in wartime. The protagonist in pathographies such as these is frequently a football or soccer player, sometimes a runner (Morris, Lund, Buchanan). These books often seem close to eulogies: their purpose is to commend these culture-heroes and, in so doing, to celebrate the sportsmanlike qualities perceived as making them heroes.[9] Thus Brian Piccolo, fullback for the Chicago Bears, is described in Jeannie Morris's pathography as having "the heart of a giant and that rare form of courage that allows him to kid himself and his opponent—cancer" (163). Piccolo is twenty-six years old when he is diagnosed as having a rare form of cancer—embryonal cell carcinoma in the chest cavity. He dies from this six months later. Throughout the pathography, he is presented as cheerful, courageous, humorous, and eminently likeable. If he sometimes felt or behaved in a less than admirable way, we are not told of it. This athlete-patient always seems to be on the playing field.

In William Buchanan's *A Shining Season*, John Baker, a twenty-four-year-old runner in training for the Olympics who develops embryonal cell cancer, similarly demonstrates the heroism often associated with a star athlete. The pathography describes the first ominous symptom of Baker's disease (a tendency to fall while running), next his discovery of a lump on his testicle leading to exploratory surgery that reveals widespread malignancy, and then his treatment: surgical removal of cancerous nodes, chemotherapy, and radiation. Baker's heroism becomes most pronounced as the end of his life draws near: he releases his fiancée, not by telling her that he has terminal cancer, but by intimating that the relationship is not working out; he refuses pain-killing medication until the pain becomes unendurable; and he devotes his remaining months to being an outstanding athletic coach for teenagers, going out of his way to make those last days "count."

A more recent pathography is Dave Dravecky's *Comeback* (1990), a book prefaced with endorsements by Ronald Reagan and George Bush. A pitcher for a major league baseball team, Dravecky develops a swelling on his arm—his pitching arm—that turns out to be a malignant tumor. He undergoes surgery to remove the tumor, also most of the deltoid muscle and some of the humerus; and he is told by his doctors that he will never play baseball again. But determination and hard work defy medical predictions, and six months later he pitches a winning game, though he breaks his arm in doing so. The dramatic center of the book is not the operation but his "comeback"—the Big Game with its wildly cheering fans. Similarly, the theme of the book is not so much his cancer as his attempts to overcome any limitation caused by the disease. As he observes in a later book, "when I was out there on the mound in my comeback game, I wasn't out there alone. I was out there with every other person who had faced adversity and who had the opportunity to overcome it" (1992, 194). Like the earlier pathographies about Brian Piccolo and John Baker, this is a simple, direct book—a contrast to the many bizarre or angry pathographies published around the same time. Dravecky is always brave and determined; never fearful, morose, or complaining. He is a "good" patient, and his attitude toward his doctors, therapies, and hospitalization is uniformly positive. This star athlete is a symbol of the drive always to "keep on playing." Thus he resists in every way he can the inevitable retirement from baseball that his illness forces on him, remarking: "It was an instinct. No matter what, you keep on. That had been my motto. Be a tiger. Never give up" (1990, 240).

Other pathographies extend the myth of the athlete to ordinary citizens. These narratives tend to be more complicated and nuanced. Though they celebrate the sportsmanship that is so highly valued in American culture, they also document some of the private and more negative aspects of a serious illness—the anger, despair, and sense of guilt that do not fit the image of the star athlete. An example is Herbert Howe's *Do Not Go Gentle,* where we encounter an elaborate formulation of the sports metaphor. A thirty-one-year-old student with a rare form of fibrosarcoma and a twenty-percent chance of survival, Howe deals with both his illness and its disabling treatment procedures by turning to sports—swimming, boxing, running, canoeing, squash, weight lifting. The result is that what began as a mild interest becomes an obsession: cancer, he realizes, "transformed my life into a sports analogy" (180). Howe's pathography

ends with his entering a canoe race—not any ordinary canoe race but the
world's championship. He emphasizes that his aim in entering is not to
win, yet because the race symbolizes for him "resistance and endurance"
(167), the aim really *is* to win. The canoe itself is an appropriate symbol
for a body damaged by disease—he refers to it as a clearly inferior model,
an "80-pound clunker"—and Howe's determination to race against
lighter and sleeker models represents an attitude toward his illness that
is not denial but a refusal to allow the inferior vessel, the life or body
damaged by disease, to interfere with "the race."

As this pathography demonstrates, the paradigm of the patient as athlete celebrates those sportsmanlike qualities that our culture generally
admires, especially in a context of crisis: courage, a sense of fair play, self-
reliance, and most important, the determination to win and the ability
to lose. For Howe, these attitudinal myths do indeed serve an enabling
function. But embedded within this pathography is another story, a mi-
croform of the genre that negatively dramatizes these same attitudes. This
is the brief pathography of Paula Williams, who is dying of cancer, and
her husband, who feels that she should try to fight her illness. Howe encounters them both during one of his hospitalizations. Williams rebukes
his wife for taking the pain-killers she obviously needs and reproaches her
for "giving in," pointing to Howe as exemplifying the results of a positive attitude and a fighting spirit. Only a few days before she dies—and
this woman is by now enduring great suffering—Williams laments her
negativity, remarking that "if Paula gives in now, both she and I'll lose
respect for her. . . . These are her last days. They're her final chance to
show everybody what a really fine person she is" (143).

The inclusion of this vignette of Paula Williams, who would seem to
be victimized by the same attitude that has facilitated Howe's recovery,
saves this pathography from the shallow optimism that sometimes characterizes others. The mere fact of its inclusion acknowledges the problematic aspect of the athletic paradigm—the idea that the ill person is
obligated to perform for an audience, to undertake publicly some feat of
courage or endurance.

In many ways, the paradigm of the athlete resembles the military
myth. Indeed, the analogy between war and game may be the result of
an actual kinship between them long ago: for example, there are funeral
games in the *Iliad* and the *Aeneid* which are quite clearly a ritual enact-
ment of the same skills required of the soldier in warfare. Both paradigms

celebrate courage and self-reliance, both disallow dependency, passivity, and self-pity, and both share the sense that recovering from an illness is like winning a battle or an athletic contest—"beating" an adversary, or the odds, or both.

The differences between the two paradigms are more subtle. Under the martial metaphor, illness is seen as a battle between the forces of life and death. But in the athletic analogy, the illness becomes not so much an enemy to be defeated as a challenge to be confronted, an obstacle to be overcome. Moreover, the metaphor of illness as war is to some extent delusory, as Judith Wilson Ross observes, since it implies that "somehow victory lies ahead" (42). The truth is, of course, that death's inevitability forecloses any chance of victory: though individual battles may be won, the war is one we all will lose. But it is also true that the power of the metaphor may stem in part from what J. R. R. Tolkien, in his famous essay on *Beowulf,* calls the "paradox of defeat inevitable yet unacknowledged"—the sense of perfect courage displayed in a battle that is fated to be lost. Here the athletic paradigm is very different, as the focus is not really on the adversary at all; instead, it is on the *self* in its struggle to recover from illness. So athletes are frequently trained to focus not on the opposing team or on the runner or swimmer whose time they are trying to beat, but on themselves, on perfecting their own skills, whether of strength or speed or dexterity. In the athletic analogy, then, the individual's only real opponent is his or her own limitations.

One of the most important differences between the paradigms of soldier and athlete is the difference between war, which is always seen as serious, and sports, which by nature belong to the realm of "play" or "game"—an autotelic construct with an invented set of objectives and rules created for pleasure and entertainment. There is an irony to the idea that illness is like athletics, because even the professional athlete always has an alternate life, a "real" life not governed by the rules of the game. He or she always has the option of leaving the field, walking out of the game, taking off the uniform, and going home. Perhaps part of the success of this particular paradigm for many ill people is this element of wish-fulfillment—the defiant assertion that illness is like a game and that in the game of cancer or AIDS there will be a terminus, and at the end, when the game or the illness is over, the player or patient will simply return to an ordinary life in "the real world."

The Journey Myth

In general, the journey motif is less fully realized in pathography than the military myth, perhaps because its less aggressive, quieter, and more introverted ethos does not appeal to our contemporary fascination with power and force. But the journey remains a potent and ancient metaphor for any kind of heroic exploration of the unknown, the dangerous, and the frightening and is thus especially appropriate to experiences of serious illness.

This myth can take several forms. One is the familiar quest motif, where the hero journeys into distant lands, undergoes various ordeals and trials, and returns with some gift or trophy. The analogy here with illness and pathography is evident. Like Aeneas descending into the Underworld or Perceval in pursuit of the Holy Grail, the protagonist in a pathography often appears as a hero who ventures into the perilous otherworld of illness and death and returns to the realm of the ordinary with some prize or knowledge.

The counterpart in pathography to the faraway realm to which the mythic hero must travel is the hospital. As so often happens, metaphor here is rooted in literal fact, the mythic in actual experience. To go from home to hospital is to make a journey: however long or short that journey may be, the psychic distance is immense. The individual—now a patient—crosses a threshold into a strange otherworld of rituals and ordeals, an unknown territory that must be negotiated alone and, often, in pain and fear. One can have the same sense of crossing a threshold—though on a smaller scale—in entering a doctor's office or examining room; one experiences something of the same change of worlds simply in becoming bedridden. The bed itself becomes a "sickbed," perhaps even a "deathbed"; the spouse or parent or adult child turns into a caregiver; the whole rhythm, pattern, and purpose of life drastically alters; even the body—that most intimate and familiar of the worlds in which we live—is transformed. Illness is like the hero's call to adventure, only this is a call that cannot be refused: whether they want to or not, the sick become denizens of a strange land.

In the mythic paradigm of the heroic journey, there is usually something gained from the hero's otherworldly travels that is brought back to the everyday world. This prize may be as concrete as the Golden Fleece secured by Jason and his Argonauts, the Golden Apples of the Hesperides brought back by Herakles, and the plant of eternal youthfulness secured by Gilgamesh; or as abstract as the Arthurian knights' vision of the Holy Grail and the understanding of the future that Aeneas brings back from his sojourn in Hades.[10] But what is the counterpart in pathography to the object of the quest, the prize the mythic hero brings back with him? The patient may simply return with the gift of health or life renewed—however temporarily—in the remission of disease. Or the sick person may bring back the gift of knowledge, that vision of a deeper meaning in life that serious illness or impending death sometimes confers upon the sick and that sometimes leads to profound personal changes. This alteration in oneself and in one's vision of life is common to both the myths of journey and of rebirth; the two myths differ in that rebirth is transformational whereas the journey is developmental, and the change effected is less dramatic and more subtle.

In another sense, the prize brought back from a sojourn in the "kingdom of the sick" may be seen as the pathography itself, the record of an experience articulated, shaped, and formulated. The patient who writes a pathography is like long-suffering, wise Odysseus—who is and is not the same Odysseus who set out from Troy—telling the story of his adventures to Alkinoös or Penelope. In the *Odyssey*, what Odysseus went through and what he learned from it are not separated. In the act of telling his story, experience and its meaning come together. The same is true in a pathography: the gift of wisdom these survivors bring back is implicit in their whole experience and communicated to us in its retelling.

A variant of the journey myth is the theme of exile. Unlike the quest, exile is involuntary and evokes feelings of estrangement, alienation, and separation. The exile is condemned to wander in strange and foreign territories; the quester seeks them out. In a sense, the difference is one of perspective: the exile yearns for what has been left behind; the quester looks forward to the unknown that lies ahead. The myth of exile aptly expresses the way certain kinds of illness are experienced. Historically, those afflicted with plague or infectious illnesses who are ritually excluded from human society conform to this archetype. In the past, the leper was the archetypal exile; today, AIDS (and to a lesser extent, cancer) carries the stigma of contagion. Unlike the quest motif, in the myth of exile there is no "return" to the ordinary world. As one might expect, it is in the AIDS pathography that one is most likely to find the myth of exile.

Another variant of the journey myth is the passage into the realm of the dead—an archetype associated with such figures as Christ in the Harrowing of Hell, Orpheus in his descent into Hades to recover Eurydice, or Aeneas in his Underworld pilgrimage to meet his father, Anchises. In pathography, this expression of the myth is not as frequent as the others; when it appears, it does so most often in the context of open-heart surgery. And this is not surprising, given our habit of associating death and the cessation of the heartbeat. Indeed, the most vivid expressions of the death-journey are the accounts of "after-life" experiences, which are quite literally journeys into death and back.

Finally, the journey myth is a construct for human mentation itself—the capacity of the exploring mind, especially the imagination, to transcend a given condition by achieving understanding of and mastery over it. In many pathographies, the journey myth is tacit—a myth alluded to and drawn upon rather than developed and utilized fully. Thus there are a surprising number of pathographies whose titles or subtitles evoke the journey archetype: *Climbing toward the Light: A Journey of Growth, Understanding and Love; The Doctor/The Patient: The Personal Journey of a Physician with Cancer; Mind, Fantasy and Healing: One Woman's Journey from Conflict and Illness to Wholeness and Health; Coming Back: One Man's Journey to the Edge of Eternity and Spiritual Rediscovery; Voyage and Return;* and *Beyond AIDS: A Journey into Healing.* These titles attract potential readers by suggesting all the various meanings associated with the journey myth. Whether they originate with author or publisher, they allude to what is at the core of the experience: they appeal to the reader precisely because they promise that what seems frightening, confusing, and devoid of meaning will be resolved into a reassuring and empowering pattern. The energies of the journey myth are drawn upon by such overt allusions as these titles, but the whole of the narrative can also be seen as following the shape of the myth. What at one level is a linear succession of discrete events—both ordinary and traumatic—is organized into a progressive pattern that reaches toward personal growth or deeper insight. The quest motif resonates with this effort.

The use of the journey theme as pathographical formulation varies from intuitive, half-conscious allusion to highly articulated mythology. For some authors, the journey is actually perceived as one into death and back. Bernice Kavinoky in her pathography characterizes her experience with cancer as a "voyage and return." James L. Johnson perceives his heart surgery as an occasion "to face squarely into death and make one of the most revolutionary journeys of my life . . . over and back" (Prologue). Esther Goshen-Gottstein, waiting for her husband to come out of a coma (despite medical predictions), likens her alternating hope and despair to the voices of Telemachus and Athena in the *Odyssey,* awaiting Odysseus' return. Realizing "that I had to find the appropriate metaphor by which to live," she uses the journey metaphor to sustain her through this period: "'Moshe has gone on a journey but has not informed us when he will return.' Here was both the indeterminate future and my hope for Moshe's return" (32, 33).

Other pathographers see the journey not as one into the realm of death but as one that explores the inner world of the psyche. In her pathography about cancer, Alice Hopper Epstein observes: "The process of regaining my health sent me on a fascinating journey into my mind"(vii). Her husband, a psychologist who acts as her therapist and who has written the introduction to her book, discovers that what he knows about the mind here proves inadequate: his "map," he writes, is "insufficient for charting the course" (xiv).

For yet other authors, the journey is one into the realm of the disease itself. Neurologist Oliver Sacks likens himself as a doctor to an explorer of "the furthest Arctics and Tropics of neurological disorder" (1984, 110). But when he himself experiences a neurological complaint that he does not understand and his physicians refuse to acknowledge, he faces "a chartless land" and feels as though he "had fallen off the map, the world, of the knowable" (110–11). In more general terms, Susan Sontag describes all sickness as an "emigrat[ion] to the kingdom of the ill" (1979, 3). Sontag's metaphor of the ill person's "more onerous citizenship" in the kingdom of the sick is quoted by Le Anne Schreiber in her pathography about her mother's illness and death from cancer (70). It is of interest that Schreiber, deeply immersed in the world of sickness as she cares for her dying mother, identifies herself as sharing, though vicariously, this "more onerous citizenship." She writes of her sense of the gulf between herself and those belonging to the world of the living: "We inhabited different planets, breathed a different atmosphere" (268). In similar fashion, Paul Monette in *Borrowed Time* repeatedly uses the image of being an exile "on the moon" to refer to the sense of radical separateness and alienation from the everyday world experienced by AIDS sufferers. Robert Murphy also uses the theme of exile in *The Body Silent,* elaborating the theme in comparing his spinal cord disease to an "extended anthropological field trip" (ix). An anthropologist and a quadriplegic, Murphy's primary focus is not his medical experience but the social milieu created by extreme physical disability. Thus he observes, following the conceit of the anthropological field trip: "Through [illness and disability] I have sojourned in a social world no less strange to me at first than those of the Amazon forests" (ix).

In all these varied examples illness and disability seem to have generated a separate world, one with a very different set of rules and routines, values and goals. Those pathographers who describe illness as a world apart do so like early European explorers writing about the "new World"—as something surprising, terrible, wonderful. But to reach the world of illness, one need not traverse sea or jungle; this world lies just beneath the apparently safe surface of the phenomenal world. This image of illness as a separate world is striking as evidence of the extent to which serious illness and death have been excluded from "ordinary" life. As Sacks observes, following an extended recovery from a leg injury, "I have since had a deeper sense of the horror and wonder which lurk behind life and which are concealed, as it were, behind the usual surface of health" (14).

Arnold Mandell's pathography is an elaborate meditation on the journey myth that coalesces with the myth of rebirth. Entitled *Coming of Middle Age, a Journey,* this book consists of Mandell's reflections on his life seen from the perspective of a coronary intensive care unit. Mandell, who is both a neuroscientist and a practising psychoanalyst, uses the concepts and terminology of neuroscience to write about the transition he hopes to make—a transition that he sees as a journey—from a life of extroversion and competitiveness to a life of inwardness and detachment. The core of the book is his idea of "a path from death in the first cycle into a fresh second cycle" (111). The journey motif appears here as a vehicle for the myth of rebirth—a rebirth out of the "first-cycle issues of the middle-brain," which includes such activities as growing up, getting married, having children—and into a "second cycle" where contemplation, quiet, and detachment are most important.

In each of these pathographies, the author appears to be drawing upon the journey theme as a part of his or her cultural legacy and perhaps as a repository of lost collective rituals. In all cases, even Sontag's, it would appear to be an enabling myth. Not only does the journey serve as a formulation of the experience, a way to organize the dramatic changes that accompany a serious illness; but in its archaic connotations of heroism and courage, the journey motif, like the military myth, restores to the ill person a sense of personal dignity and social value.

Most of these pathographies use the myth in a more or less casual manner; they do not explore and elaborate its deeper implications. An exception is Oliver Sacks's *A Leg to Stand On.* Sacks here describes a leg injury, incurred while hiking in Norway but attended to in a British hospital.

Though the injury is repaired by surgery, Sacks's recovery is not what he or the medical staff anticipate. Instead, he experiences a profoundly unsettling disturbance of body image: not only does he lose all sensation in his leg but he also loses recognition that the leg "belongs" to him. This proprioceptive impairment is all the more difficult because his physician refuses to acknowledge it.

The journey myth is the organizing metaphor of Sacks's pathography. It is first suggested (or perhaps reinforced) by the casual comments of one of the doctors Sacks confronts during the early days of his experience, who soothes him with the remark: "Take it easy! The whole thing, going through it, is really a pilgrimage" (113). It is a comment that Sacks mentions over and over in the course of his narrative, and it can be seen as summarizing—or perhaps instigating—the pathographical formulation of the entire experience.

The time he spends as a patient does turn out to be very much like a pilgrimage, a journey into a mental landscape that he initially experiences as "limbo." His passage through this state blends the three realms of the *Divine Comedy* with the dark night of the soul in Saint John of the Cross: by giving way to "an intense and absolute and essential passivity," the Hell of his physical and psychological condition is transformed into a Purgatory that he experiences as a kind of holy darkness, and that opens out into a radiant secret sense of God and "a curious, paradoxical joy" (108–12). Sacks's illness has become a Dantean "journey of the soul" in which he "journey[s] to despair and back" (113).[11] In Dante, however, the pilgrim-author is accompanied through the realms of Hell, Purgatory, and Heaven first by Virgil and then by Beatrice. But Sacks's pilgrimage is marked by the absence of the Dantean figure of the guide. Indeed, it is his physicians' refusal to acknowledge Sacks's own subjective experience after the operation—lack of sensation and the absence of a proprioceptive sense of the leg—that is the cause of Sacks's despair, his "dark night of the soul." The doctor who is able to relate to his or her patients, acknowledge their feelings, empathize with them and give comfort to them, inevitably takes on the mantle of the "guide" of legend and folklore. But rarely in pathographies is the physician in fact represented as acting as guide for the ill person. Indeed, one author uses the metaphor of the journey to comment on the damage done by doctors who neglect their patients' emotional life: "The failure to provide safe conduct is the most serious shortcoming in cancer treatment today" (Graham, 66).

In Sacks's pathography, the failure of his physician "to provide safe conduct" is carefully anatomized and recorded. Sacks tries to explain his condition to his doctor, feels that he is being ignored, and goes so far as to accuse him of not listening. The doctor responds: "No, indeed, I can't waste time with 'experiences' like this. I'm a practical man, I have work to do." The dialogue continues as follows:

Sacks: "Experience aside then, the leg doesn't *work*."

Doctor: "That's not my business."

Sacks: "Then whose business is it? Specifically, there is something physiologically the matter. What about a neurological opinion, nerve-conduction tests, EMGs, etc.?" (107)

The dialogue ends with the doctor turning away without answering. Sacks describes the confrontation later on as concluding in a tacit agreement not to allude again to this dimension of his experience—to the "deeper things."

But Sacks is able to confront the failure of his physicians to provide safe conduct by finding substitutes. Abandoned by his doctor, he turns to literature and finds his "guide" in the writings of the Old Testament Psalmist, John Donne, T. S. Eliot, Dante, Saint John of the Cross, and Nietzsche. Sacks's own pathography must be seen as a part of this tradition. Like Eliot in *The Wasteland,* Sacks finds a basic mythic pattern refracted in a range of literary sources, all of which interact to interpret and direct his experience. These writings become the guide he lacks, and his own book can be seen as offering to serve this same function for others.[12]

In this pathography, the journey myth is clearly enabling. But implicit in Sacks's success is an explanation for the potential failure of this myth for others. In the exchange that Sacks so carefully describes (quoted above), the doctor fails because he cannot bring himself to face "deeper things," and Sacks's passage out of limbo and back "to light and life" is accomplished by recourse to poetry and religion. Sacks succeeds in his pilgrimage—he emerges from the Hell in which he finds himself—because of his unusual intelligence and his formidable mastery of great literature. But most individuals do not share these gifts, nor are they themselves physicians, as is Sacks. This suggests that for the individual who does not have Sacks's resources, the failure of a doctor to listen—to acknowledge his or her patient's actual experience and to confront those "deeper things"—may have far-reaching consequences.

A second way in which the journey myth is manifested in Sacks's pathography is the similarity between his experience and what anthropologists call rites of passage. These rites signify the transition from one state or condition of life to another, such as the initiation rites accompanying the transition from childhood to puberty, installation rites signifying the transition from ordinary citizenship to king or religious leader, and also funeral ceremonies and marriages. The ethnographer Arnold van Gennep, the anthropologist Victor Turner, and mythographers Mircea Eliade and Joseph Campbell discuss the rite of passage as marked by three phases. The first phase is that of separation and involves actions whereby the individual, whom Turner nicely refers to as "the passenger," undergoes a detachment from his or her position and relationships (also his or her rights and responsibilities) in the world. The second phase is one of transition or marginality—a liminal state where the individual "passes through a cultural realm that has few or none of the attributes of the past or coming state" (Turner, 94). The third phase is one of aggregation or incorporation, when individuals return to the world they have left, reassuming prior status, rights, and relationships or assuming new ones.

In his pathography, Sacks describes an experience that precisely parallels a rite of passage—a passage from the world of health into and then back out of the world of sickness. His description of the degradation, humiliation, and "systematic depersonalization" of hospital admission procedures—a description echoed in many pathographies—suggests that these procedures may be *primarily* ritual and only secondarily practical and necessary. If this is so, then hospital admission rituals serve as rites of passage conveying the sick person into the realm of illness. Sacks describes in great detail the way a person is systematically transformed into a patient. His clothes are replaced with an anonymous hospital shift, the obligatory identification bracelet substitutes a number for his name, institutional rules and regulations now govern everything that he does and that is done to him, and he discovers that the full and perhaps only explanation for certain medical activities is simply that they are "standard procedure." Other pathographers flesh out the picture of the rites of patienthood in the United States with other details: the ritual of the admitting office, where forms are completed and the patient-to-be is screened to verify insurance coverage; the obligatory wheelchair to convey patients into and out of their proper places in the hospital; the X-ray and blood tests that are so often administered routinely—meaning ritually—to patients upon admittance.

Sacks compares the process to being a prisoner or a beginning student: "One is no longer a free agent; one no longer has rights; one is no longer in the world-at-large" (46). But he also comes to see all these rites of patienthood as necessary, though the necessity is a ritual one: being in the hospital, Sacks observes, reduces an individual to a kind of "moral infancy" appropriate to "the biological and spiritual needs of the hurt creature" (165). This recognition is an important element in the journey myth (with its overtones of a rite of passage) that is central to Sacks's formulation of his experience.

Patienthood is precisely analogous to the second phase of "liminality" discussed by van Gennep and Turner, a state characterized by the three primary attributes of passivity, humility, and near-nakedness. "Liminal entities," observes Turner, are ritually dressed in such a way as to signify that they have no status and no property. Moreover, their dress makes them indistinguishable from their fellow initiates. Their behavior is expected to be both passive and humble—"they must obey their instructors implicitly, and accept arbitrary punishment without complaint" (95). Turner interprets the meaning of these ritual degradations as follows: "It is as though they are being reduced or ground down to a uniform condition to be fashioned anew and endowed with additional powers to enable them to cope with their new station in life" (95). Furthermore, the state of liminality is one where the initiate, regressed to an earlier state, will have to endure various trials and ordeals. It often involves physical mutilations of one kind or another—circumcision, subincision, extraction of an incisor—as the novice is introduced into "the mystery of blood." The result of these "sanguinary mutilations," writes Eliade, is that the novice is reborn, "radically regenerated" (28). With surprisingly few changes, these conditions are those generally expected of hospital patients today: passivity, near-nakedness, obedience, anonymity, and sometimes painful and invasive medical tests and procedures.

As we have seen, liminality is experienced by Sacks as a state he calls "limbo"—a terrifying "scotoma," a metaphysical emptiness where, imprisoned in a "roomless room" and confused by a sense of his body that his doctor refuses to acknowledge, he feels alone, disoriented, and alienated. Sacks's description of his need to relinquish his active self and assume a stance of passivity is an eloquent description of liminality: "I found this humiliating, at first, a mortification of my self—the active, masculine, ordering self, which I had equated with my science, my self-respect, my mind" (111). It is with Sacks's acceptance of this passivity that his sense of regeneration begins, and with this, he is able to perceive the whole experience as a "dark night of the soul," a holy darkness, a journey of the soul to despair and back (111–14).

The third phase, the return to the world, is in Sacks's pathography ritually structured, with recovery as "a 'pilgrimage,' a journey, in which one moved, if one moved, stage by stage, or by stations" (160–61). He describes his recovery in spatial imagery consistent with the journey metaphor dominating the pathography: each literal move to a new room or place is accompanied by an existential movement out of the contracted world of illness and into a new and wider dimension. This spatial dimension is marked by a graduated sense of expansion and freedom. So Sacks observes that "the essence of getting better" is in "emerging from self-absorption, sickness, patienthood, and confinement, to the spaciousness of health, of full being, of the real world" (156). The fact that Sacks spends several more weeks in a convalescent home reinforces the ritual aspects of his return to the world of the well. He sees this space and time as bridging the gap between sickness and health, as an "in-between" place that serves existential as well as medical needs.

In Sacks's case, the return appears to be facilitated to some extent by the nature of his injury: limbs can heal completely, which is what happens here. But for the patient with chronic illness, the return to the real world is usually a qualified one, compromised by the temporary status of remission, blurred by the need to accommodate an ongoing medical condition, or conditioned by mutilating therapies. Thus one pathographer writes about the difficulty experienced by a typical cancer patient: "He has been to the brink, and he feels he is still clinging to the precipice. He has no idea how to reenter the world he left behind" (Graham, 91). In such a situation, the journey metaphor can prove genuinely helpful, since it not only acknowledges the sense of estrangement and "otherness" felt by so many patients, but it also can provide formulae for the return to ordinary life. Indeed, the individual who experiences his or her illness as a journey into the depths of life, or death, can return to the ordinary world with an empowering sense of the deeper meaning of things.

Battle and Journey Compared

Of the two myths we have examined, the military myth is clearly the more prominent in pathography: it occurs with greater frequency and tends to be more consciously utilized and fully elaborated than the journey myth. Several reasons can be suggested as to why this is so. To begin with, the military myth connotes power and aggressive action and, thus, serves as a strong contrast to the passivity usually associated with an illness. Etymologically, "patient" and "passive" come from same root, the Latin verb meaning to suffer or endure. A "patient" is also the opposite of an "agent," in that the latter acts and the former is acted upon. Those who are seriously ill in our society become patients in both senses—persons who must passively endure not only the disease but also what is done for and to them. The military myth is the antidote to a passivity now widely assumed to be deleterious not only to a patient's morale but even to his or her health. Perhaps the military myth is so frequent in pathographies about AIDS because of these associations with power, action, and a refusal to be victimized. Moreover, the myth of illness as warfare is syntonic with many of the constructs of medicine, whereas that of the journey is often not. As we have seen demonstrated in the pathographies of Ryan and Sacks, it is easier for physicians to play the role of a "general" in the war against disease than it is for them to succeed as a "guide" leading the patient on the journey into and back out of the world of sickness.

The military myth fulfills all three of the functions we have ascribed to myth in general. It is integrative, gathering up the many phenomena of an illness experience—the enemy disease; the army of doctors, nurses, and other medical personnel; the whole armamentarium of therapies—and subsuming them into the master metaphor of warfare. It is connective, implicitly situating the individual struggle with personal illness within the larger war against cancer or AIDS. And it is analogical, in that all such mythic warfare is conceived as a struggle of good against evil, light against darkness, life against death.

Though the journey myth is not as broadly represented or as deeply realized in pathography, it too has potential as an enabling myth, though in rather different ways. If the military myth is confrontational, realized in strategies planned and executed for defeating an enemy, the journey myth is linear, realized in a metaphorical movement away from and back into the everyday world. Moreover, this movement is often one with spiritual overtones: when patients return from their experience in the "otherworld" of illness, they return *changed* by that experience. The military myth tends to be medically syntonic. But in its concern with spiritual or developmental aspects of a sickness, the journey myth tends to be if not medically dystonic, certainly medically irrelevant—epiphenomenal to the nature and purpose of treatment. Another difference between the two is that the military myth better allows for community. In Ryan's pathography, his physicians, nurses, and technicians are a part of the "war effort," and his many friends are compared to members of the Resistance movement. The journey myth tends to be more privatistic, emphasizing the aloneness and isolation of the patient entering "the kingdom of the sick." Of course this isolation is not total in either the myth or the illness experience: the hero who descends to the underworld has a guide, Greek heroes are often aided directly by the gods, the knight on a quest is supported by his squire, the adventurer in a fairy-tale encounters helpful animals and magical allies— and all these have their obvious medical counterparts. But in essence the journey myth in pathography is an inner experience, one usually unaided by physician or friend.

Pathographies that deploy the journey myth often do so allusively, unlike many of the pathographies organized around the military myth. Sacks's work is unusual in this respect, in that he shows how it is possible to turn a latent archetype into one that is rich, full, dynamic, humanly functional, and even—in its own way—medically syntonic. Much that is negative or confusing in the illness experience makes sense in the metaphoric perspective Sacks provides. For Sacks demonstrates that the painful ordeals and humiliating routines of the hospital can take on meaning and purpose if they are perceived as a rite of passage, initiating patients into the world of sickness and ushering them back out of it again. In opening this perspective, Sacks, whose own lack of a guide is so crucial to his experience, becomes a guide to others.

The journey and the battle myths, so often associated in legend and mythology, are in pathography complementary ways of formulating an experience of illness; in addition, they are myths that both perceive and create meaning. They help us see what is actually as well as metaphorically true: that the struggle against disease really *is* like a war as microbes are killed or cancerous cells destroyed, that the compassionate physician really *is* a guide in the patient's journey through the world of illness, and that the short passage from the recovery room or intensive care unit to a private room or public ward really *is* a journey back toward life. As creations, both myths help turn an experience where one is primarily acted upon into one where one can act—precisely by giving it meaning. Pathographers who use these myths, whether they merely allude to them or whether they consciously explore and elaborate them, are participating in this double process of perceiving and creating meaning. Such mythic formulations of illness are empowering: the ill person understands the way sickness is like a war or a journey into a distant country; but at the same time he or she is *choosing* to give that meaning to it, and this is an act of creative choice in an area of life where choice and creativity are almost wholly denied.[13]

CHAPTER FOUR

✦

Constructing Death: Myths about Dying

Pathographies of death and dying are a part of the efflorescence in the past two decades of books about this subject—books that range from learned psychological, sociological, and medical analyses to how-to-deal-with-death manuals. Side by side with these writings are the plays, stories, novels, and television and film dramas that depict what it is like to have a terminal illness or to lose a child, a spouse, a parent, or a lover. The appearance of all this literature is itself a striking reversal of the relative paucity of writings about death in the first half of the twentieth century. If for an earlier generation death was a taboo, for us it seems to border on an obsession.

Aristotle observed long ago in the *Nichomachean Ethics* that "death is the most terrible of all things" (III.5, 975). But today, with the possibility that one's life might be prolonged indefinitely, this statement takes on a new meaning: what many now fear is a "medical death"—the technological prolongation of life at the expense of any real sense of the quality of life. And indeed, both scholarly and popular writings concur that medical technology has far outstripped our ability, as a culture, to know how to use it wisely. Certainly it is unwise to regard death as "an enemy to be conquered," an attitude that Robert Veatch sees as the result of both our "activist approach" to life and our recent technological ability to control biological processes (15–18). The report of the pathographer confirms the theories of the scholar. So Peter Noll, diagnosed as having cancer of the bladder, defends his decision to reject surgical intervention: "I don't want to get caught in the surgical-urological-radiological machine because then I'll lose my freedom piecemeal, my will will be broken as hope diminishes, and I'll end up one way or another in the well-known death room that everyone skirts" (5).

One might interpret our recent interest in death and dying as evidence that, as a culture, we have arrived at our own understanding of death—a "death-myth" for our time. In support of this idea, David Duclow writes that Broadway plays in the 1970s (*Whose Life Is It Anyway?* and *The Shadow Box*) show that the values and practices of the death-and-dying movement are coming to function as "a contemporary equivalent to the traditional *ars moriendi.*" Culturally, he observes, "an art of dying is in the making," one which "includes a renewed emphasis on truth-telling, the values of autonomy and control, a myth outlining the journey of death, and rituals of terminal care" (199, 212). Duclow's argument seems convincing not only when we examine "dying on Broadway" but also when we reflect on the continuing popularity of Kübler-Ross's *On Death and Dying*, first published in 1969.

Pathography, however, points to quite a different conclusion. Pathographies written over the past thirty years that describe the illness and death of a loved one suggest not that a new *ars moriendi* shaped by the death-and-dying movement is under way but that we are still in search of a model for "the good death." The sheer variety of models formulated for the good death in these narratives suggests that there is no one emergent art of dying; instead, there seem to be almost as many versions of an art of dying as there are books about dying. As Larry Churchill points out, "Each [person] is as unique and individual in dying as in living" (33). Eric Robinson in his pathography indicates skepticism about glib acceptance of Kübler-Ross's formulae: "Death is a personal experience and each one of us should be allowed to die his or her death and not be expected to conform to some general pattern" (ix). The recent concern with death and dying may signal not the emergence of a new art of dying but a desperate cultural search for helpful models of "how" to die.

Medieval and Renaissance Christian cultures, with their *ars moriendi* tradition, had certain prescribed rituals for death—practices that reflected the belief in an afterlife—as well as the conviction that bodily illness may reflect an underlying spiritual sickness, that the good Christian's life should be an imitation of the life and death of Christ, and that "right living" entails a good measure of thinking about death. The graveyard scene where Hamlet meditates on death, holding the skull of "poor Yorick" in his hands, stems from this tradition; so also does Walton's vivid account of John Donne, posing for his portrait in a winding-sheet and in the posture of death, which portrait he had put by his bedside "where it continued and became his hourly object till his death" (52).

The works that stemmed from the *ars moriendi* tradition were guidebooks to the art of dying, manuals of instruction for those facing death. This genre can be traced back as far as the early fifteenth century, with Jean de Gerson's *Opusculum Tripartitium* and the anonymous *Tractatus* or *Speculum, Artis Bene Moriendi*. The *Tractatus* was an immensely popular treatise that soon became known all over Europe through its various secular translations. In England, the genre underwent further development with the introduction of Stoic themes in the Renaissance; it was modified in the late sixteenth century with the rise of Calvinism and then the Counter-Reformation, and reached its peak in the seventeenth-century Jeremy Taylor's much-admired *The Rule and Exercises of Holy Dying* (Beaty; Kastenbaum 1989). Though the handbooks representative of these different eras vary greatly, spanning as they do 250 years of Christian history, they share certain repeated themes and practices: the recognition that dying is both difficult and fearful; a set of verbal formulae and ritual practices to help the dying person—called *Moriens*—die "well and surely" by strengthening his or her faith; the presence of a priest or pastor to direct *Moriens* in the recitation of prayers and "obsecrations" as well as in the performance of various rituals at the proper time; and provision for a group of bystanders who offer spiritual assistance of various sorts.

It is not only in Christian cultures that one finds an *ars moriendi*, for the Stoics of the ancient world had a similarly codified set of attitudes and practices regarding death; so also did the traditional Japanese. We cannot accurately know the pressures and distortions such models may have imposed. However, it would seem that the strong emotions that arise in response to death are often more easily dealt with in the context of a broadly applicable cultural paradigm—a network of beliefs, attitudes, and practices within which dying persons, as well as those connected with their death, can negotiate this difficult rite of passage.

An *ars moriendi* is of course closely bound up with mythic conceptions of death. Indeed, death seems to be the kind of existential fact that particularly evokes myth: almost all cultures have, at least in their history, a body of myths that describe the life of the soul after death and the afterworld(s) in which the soul resides. For death marks the boundary of our knowledge as of our lives: it is the definitive expression of our limitations as human beings. Moreover, death is almost by definition an aggregate of negatives:

cessation of breathing, failure of heartbeat, loss of consciousness. To "know" death is to know negation and absence—something our minds cannot really do.

It is because death is so totally unknown but at the same time so imperatively real, for each of us, that the attempt to come to terms with it is expressed in myth. We are all familiar with the form such myths take in the West: Greek heroes of antiquity are translated after their death into constellations or dispatched to the Islands of the Blest; Germanic heroes are spirited away by the Valkyries to revel in Valhalla; and in the meritocracy of Dante's *Divine Comedy,* souls enjoy everlasting bliss in the radiance of God or endure everlasting torment in the bowels of Hell. Such myths, rather than explaining death, tend to explain it away: they seem to dissolve the reality of death even as they acknowledge it. Death may well be the Gorgon head that none of us can fully look at, and one important function of myths about dying is to deflect our gaze from death itself to a "storied" reflection.

Our modern technological culture is unusual in that it has no central, vital myth about death that can dictate an "art of dying" appropriate to the pluralistic world of twentieth-century values and medical realities. What replaces an effective cultural myth about dying is the tendency to deny death—a tendency that, paradoxically, exists side by side with our obsession with death.[1] And this pervasive ethos of denial has generated its own set of ritual practices: the hospital death behind closed curtains, the practice of spiriting a corpse out of the ward on a stretcher specially designed to conceal it, the corpse so transformed by cosmetic reconstruction as to be nearly unrecognizable. It goes without saying that practices such as these, generated out of a denial or avoidance of death, generally serve the needs neither of the dying nor of those who grieve for the dying and mourn the dead.

But the late twentieth century is not wholly cut off from other times and other ways of thought, despite the assertions of some that "postmodernism" is a world unto itself. Besides the habit of denial, we also have available to us a range of models of death from other or earlier cultures—models that survive through religion, literature, and art. Pathographies about death and dying can be seen as drawing upon these cultural or religious fragments of myth, in an uncanny fulfillment of Eliot's famous dictum in *The Wasteland:* "These fragments I have shored against my ruin." The following morphology of models for the good death—models for the

most part available to us as fragments from other cultural belief-systems—
may be helpful in understanding the particular formulations about dying
in the pathographies discussed in the remainder of this chapter.

Christianity provides what may be termed the myth of sacred death.
Death, as embodied in the crucifixion and resurrection of Christ, is transcendence and transformation. As I understand the story of the Passion, its
implicit logic is that the meaning of death emerges in the act of dying itself. Christ knows from the first that he must die, and the death he suffers
is a very real one: his physical suffering is emphasized in the emaciated
body hanging from the cross, the blood that flows from the wound in his
side and the crown of thorns, the tangled and matted hair, and the nail
marks gouged into his hands and feet; his mental suffering is realized in his
plea that God might spare him this awful ordeal and in that cry of derelic-
tion—"My God, my God, why hast thou forsaken me?" The death of
Christ preserves all the agony and terror of the ordinary human being confronting death. In this it becomes explicitly an object of imitation, as the
older *ars moriendi* tradition understood: each individual death can derive
its meaning from the greater archetype. But, most important, this agoniz-
ing "passage" can be endured because it is not final: the redeemed, in imitation of Christ, can look forward to the resurrection of the soul after the
death of the body. The idea of resurrection is in some sense a denial of
death, but it is important that, in the story of Christ, it comes after the
vividly realized death scene of the crucifixion. This mythos paradoxically
enables one to accept death fully—and accept it for the terrible and fearful thing it really is—because death has been defeated by the sacrifice of
Christ and invalidated by his bodily resurrection.

A second model is the philosophic death, the noble or "good" death
epitomized in the death of Socrates. Though Socrates believes in the immortality of the soul and in an afterlife as well, there is no explicit sense of
transcendence in this paradigm; nowhere does Socratic wisdom cross the
boundary of the sacred. Unlike Christ, Socrates thinks and talks a good
deal about the nature of death, and in fact his own death is the occasion
for a final lecture to his disciples about the immortality of the soul. The
philosophic death is accepted without fear because of the belief that death
cannot harm the just man: "The true philosopher," Socrates says to his
disciple Simmias, is "eager to die" (*Phaedo*, 9). Moreover, the true philosopher can welcome the separation of body and soul that comes with death,
since throughout his life he has worked at subjugating the passions of the

physical man to the higher passion of the love of wisdom. So Socrates observes, "Those who rightly engage in philosophy study only dying and death" (*Phaedo*, 8). A variant on the philosophic death is the Stoic suicide, best represented in the teachings and example of Seneca, whose final act was to open his veins and bleed to death in compliance with the orders of Nero.[2] Plato himself (in the *Phaedo* and *Laws*) condones suicide under certain conditions: when it is ordered by the state, when one is under the compulsion of severe pain, or when one is faced with intolerable shame. The more moderate Stoics continue this line of reasoning; others elevate suicide to a central dogma: for Seneca, suicide is of primary importance as the only truly free act possible and, thus, in and of itself ennobling. Whether Socratic or Stoic, the philosophic death is the product of reason, not emotion: it is an act whereby the individual's death can be made to express the same philosophic values that he or she lived for.

And third, there is the heroic death. The warrior's death is a pervasive theme in the mythologies of almost every culture: one thinks of the Norse Ragnarok, where heroes and gods alike join forces against the powers of darkness, or of the battlefields of Anglo-Saxon, Carolingian, or Greek epic. A particularly fine expression of the heroic ideal is a speech in the *Iliad* by "godlike Sarpedon," son of Zeus, as he goes into a battle where he is sure to die. In some of the most beautiful lines in the poem, Sarpedon exhorts his comrade into the fighting, reasoning that, since death is the fate of all, one's only choice is to die ignominiously or to die gloriously: "seeing that the spirits of death stand close about us / in their thousands, no man can turn aside nor escape them, / let us go and win glory for ourselves" (12.326–28). Here there is no transcendence or transformation, no belief in the immortality of the soul, and no promise whatsoever of an afterlife. The victory is in the courage and fearlessness with which the warrior engages in battle; death, while not a matter of indifference, is subordinate to these higher values.

These mythic paradigms of death—the sacred, the philosophic, and the heroic—illustrate the dynamic nature of myth in that each of them becomes a model for subsequent praxis. They can be (and have been) translated into practice in the various *ars moriendi* of other cultures; in our own time, in the absence of any central, coherent art of dying, they survive as fragments half-remembered and partially distorted. The discussion that follows is organized around the very different formulations arrived at by various pathographers—formulations in which one can trace elements of the paradigmatic models of sacred, philosophic, and heroic death. Previous chapters in this book have been shaped around a particular myth about illness—a "monomyth" given expression in the formulations of each author. Pathographies about dying, however, are characterized by the fragmentation of an organizing myth: the formulation each author arrives at identifies not the presence of an organizing myth but its absence. Readers may feel that at times these accounts seem forced, artificial, extreme, or even grotesque; but this impression reflects the task embraced by these authors—to create a meaningful death out of the fragments of myth available to them.

Ritual Death

Birth, puberty, marriage, death: it is around important events such as these that rituals tend to accrue. Inevitably, we seem to need to ritualize those experiences in life that evoke complex and deep responses. This need for ritual becomes problematic in a society such as our own, where for many people traditional religious belief-systems and the rituals that express those beliefs are felt to be unsatisfactory.

Hope, A Loss Survived, Richard Meryman's story of his wife's illness and death and his own experience of mourning, illustrates one way of coming to terms with this dilemma. The book is organized around what he calls "the Ritual"—his formula for the triad of illness, death, and mourning, which he believes are "a ritual as formalized as the Catholic Mass or the crowning of an English Queen" (15). The first part of the book is devoted to his wife's illness, the second part describes her slow death, and the last part concerns his mourning—a stage that he further categorizes as itself a three-stage process of "shock, pain, and grief."[3] At first glance, this division into illness, death, and mourning seems self-evident: they are so obviously phases in any such extended dying that no pattern or interpretation seems to be imposed. But at what point exactly does illness turn into dying? Are we really dealing with a process divided into clear and disjunct phases, or do the phases so blend into one another that even such an elementary division becomes an act of interpretation? Death might seem to provide an unambiguous terminus to the second phase. However, as we shall see, even Hope's death is not experienced as final by her husband.

In Meryman's pathography, the discrepancy between the actual experience and the formulation achieved in reconstruction is a difference of which the author is acutely aware. Meryman distinguishes between "the Ritual" and what he calls "the ordeal." "The Ritual" designates experience that has been ordered—assimilated, integrated, and formulated; "the ordeal" is the way he refers to the experience itself, unformulated and immediate, of his wife's illness and death. This pathography illustrates how the raw, unstructured feelings and events of "the ordeal" are transformed by the formulating idea of ritual into a series of stages, with appropriate feelings for each stage. It is as though the only way that Meryman can really grasp and endure "the ordeal" is to see it afterward as it is reflected in a clear, conceptual framework.

The pathography begins when Hope, an artist in her forties and the mother of two young girls, discovers a black mole on her back, soon diagnosed as malignant melanoma. She undergoes surgery for removal of the mole, the surrounding tissue, and the spleen. About a year later, after several operations for an enlarged eyelid, she is hospitalized again for a variety of symptoms: dizziness, numbness on the left side, and aphasia. Surgery reveals the presence of two metastatic brain tumors. For the author, this discovery marks the end of the phase of illness and the beginning of the phase of dying.

The way that Meryman perceives himself as responding to this information is worth attending to closely, for it is characteristic of the entire book: "In that moment, I began the period in the Ritual known as premourning—grieving for Hope while she was still alive, living in a limbo of last-times and too-lates without the finality of death, without the directioning sense of a mourning process under way" (102). He does not here describe exactly how he felt but, instead, invokes a category of experience, "premourning," which he then situates within its proper place in that larger abstraction, "the Ritual." The result of focusing in this way on abstract categories, phases, and stages is not only that he distances himself from painful feelings and memories but also that he obscures the sense of his wife as a person. In the narrative, Hope often seems to be sacrificed to this overall ritual formulation of the experience.

As her condition gradually deteriorates, the side-effects of her various therapies rival the symptoms of her disease in severity and number: antiseizure drugs make her feel tired and disoriented, radiation leads to loss of hair, chemotherapy results in nausea and vomiting, immunotherapy produces disfiguring obesity. Eventually her physician discovers that the cancer has metastasized to the bone marrow. Knowing that her death is both certain and imminent, Meryman decides to bring his wife home. She dies two months later.

The final part of the book concerns what Meryman calls "the mourning process" or "the mourning ritual." He does not so much describe his emotions and the events of this period in his life as refer to them—perhaps legitimize them—by abstract categories: "The complete mourning ritual, according to my reading and questioning, lasts a year and a half to two years. . . . If the first two phases are the times of surgical removal, the third is the recovery period, when you finally learn to live without the dead. The times of ease grow longer, and the sudden relapses into acute distress are fewer" (233). In passages such as this, a description of specific, personal response blends into a generalizing, prescriptive statement. What marks the change from the one to the other is often verb tense: Meryman uses past tense when he is describing actual feelings or events but present tense when he is invoking abstract categories of response. Thus he writes: "Once Hope *was* buried, I could collapse into the numbness that *marks* the first phase of mourning" or "premourning *does share* many of the mourning symptoms. At home with Hope I *was* in the state that a death *brings*." [170, 103; italics added]. The result of this kind of writing is to endow the abstract categories with a reality, a permanence, that is denied to the actual events upon which those abstractions are based.

Meryman's frequent allusions to "the Ritual" have something of this abstract quality. For ritual usually refers to a mode of behavior: it is something people do. But Meryman does not describe himself or his wife as behaving ritualistically during the events of her illness and death. Ritual in this book is an epistemological, not a descriptive term; one that suggests a mode of human understanding or feeling, not a set of fixed behaviors. In a sense, the author is using the concept of ritual here in a ritualistic way.

One function that "the Ritual" serves is as a substitute for verbal communication between Meryman and his wife. He represents them both as having tacitly agreed not to talk much about what is happening. In the initial stages of her illness, he actually withholds from Hope information about her condition, although she has indicated that she wants to know the truth and her physician sees no reason why she should not be told. His justification for doing this is linked to the role of deceiver-protector that he has created for himself: "I decided, for now, to spare Hope this dreadful prospect. I wondered if I could counterfeit optimism while burdened with secret knowledge"(45). Later on, he sees himself as helping her best by "appointing [him]self chief optimist—outwardly refusing to admit defeat, pouring reassurance into Hope" (77). At this point the reader must wonder if "Meryman" is not a symbolic name, as "Hope" clearly is.

The ultimate function of perceiving illness, death, and mourning as components of a single "Ritual" is that it enables Meryman to live beyond them. This is represented in the book's ambiguous title, *Hope, A Loss Survived*. It is a significant ambiguity, for the "loss" that Meryman survives is, literally, that of his wife; however, on a symbolic level both of them are represented in this pathography as "survivors of that loss of hope." Thus on one occasion, describing to a friend the two-year ordeal of Hope's illness and death, he concludes with the words: "'and that was how we survived'" (16). Recognizing his use of the pronoun "we," Meryman confirms that this is what indeed had happened—that, paradoxically, "on the deepest level" both of them survived the experience.

At the end of the narrative Meryman observes that an important transition in the Ritual is the "leap from survival into recovery" (236). The pathography ends with an epilogue, written during the Christmas holiday, in which the theme of survival is represented in the symbol of a Christmas tree. It is an appropriate image because it recalls Hope's death, which occurred on Christmas day four years earlier. It is also appropriate because the ritual of bringing in and decorating a live tree in midwinter—the only actual ritual in the book—symbolizes both the renewal of nature in the cycle of the seasons and also the rebirth of "hope" out of the winter of the soul. To Meryman, it signifies the goal toward which his formulation of the experience as "the Ritual" finally leads: "It is enduring the entire experience to its dregs and then turning your loss into a rebirth, into Christmas" (246).

The reference to Christmas with which Meryman concludes his book marks the way in which religious forms can survive their original meanings. What is striking about this narrative is the pervasive use of the concept of ritual in the absence of any religious belief-system. It may be significant that although Hope had been a devout Roman Catholic all her life, her religion, according to Meryman, is not very helpful to her during her illness. And his own formulation of his wife's illness and death as "the Ritual" is certainly not grounded in any particular religious belief, although it may well express a nostalgia for the comforts of orthodox religious rituals. Perhaps here the very concept of ritual as a way to understand experience serves as a substitute for the doctrines that inform religious rituals.

This is a pathography of formulation par excellence, in that the author's own particular formulation—"the Ritual"—appears to be more the subject of the book than the experience upon which it is based. In such self-referential phrases as "my mourning cure" or such universalizing statements as "the essence of mourning is gradualism," Meryman is not describing his feelings but formulating them. It is as though the focus of the book is not so much on illness, death, and mourning as it is on Meryman observing himself as he deals with these experiences. The result is that the experience itself has become a ritual: illness, death, and mourning are seen as phases of a single process, and the events and feelings appropriate to each phase are seen as orderly and purposive. Given this attitude, it is perhaps not surprising that Meryman felt it unnecessary to attend his wife's burial. For if experience *is* ritual, then rituals themselves become superfluous.

One's Own Death

A Death of One's Own, by Gerda Lerner, describes her husband's eighteen-month illness and eventual death from inoperable brain cancer. This pathography represents the attempt to impose order on experience in that process of formulation that helps people not just live through an experience but also live beyond it. Lerner's pathography differs from most, however, in that it questions the order it imposes. She sees her book as "a fragment made up of fragments. . . . a figment of the imagination, a distorted aspect of a larger whole" (7). The texture of the book effectively blends different literary modes—diary entries, poetry, autobiographical flashbacks of the author's childhood in Nazi Europe—and retrospective pathographical narrative. Both style and structure are based on a recognition of the discrepancy between actual event and remembered event; on an awareness that the "truth" of an experience blends literal realities with mythic expectations and is understood by means of modalities of description and explanation that inevitably distort as they interpret. What she offers here, she writes, is "another sort of truth: layered, organic, functional" (7).

The title of the book is taken from Rilke—"O Lord, give everyone his own death"—a title evoking the idea that the style of dying should reflect the personality of the dying person. The concept of "one's own death" suggests that death is, at least potentially, an individualized or personalized event. The idea of individualization in death is itself a remarkable reversal—a counter-myth—of the older notion of death as the great leveler, reducing king and slave alike to the same moribund status. In the literature of the medieval *ars moriendi* tradition, for example, the dying person is referred to in generalizing terms as *"Moriens"* (the dying one) or "Everyman." Appropriately, the art of dying advocated in those tracts is assumed to be universally true—adaptable to "every man." But today, the individualistic nature of death is a common assumption: thus Robert Kastenbaum and Ruth Aisenberg comment on the way death has become "decontextualized" in modern society, so that the "older system of social control" regarding aspects of death and dying is now replaced by the individual—"the individual is the primary unit now" (208)—and Phillipe Ariès observes that "Western man has come to see himself in his own death; he has discovered *la mort de soi,* one's own death" (52).

Carl Lerner is a man in his late fifties with a successful career in filmmaking. As in so many pathographies, it is during a vacation that the early symptoms of illness are first noticed: in Carl's case, stiffness of the fingers of the right hand. When he is hospitalized for diagnostic tests, a cerebral angiogram indicates the presence of a tumor on the left side of the brain. Not long thereafter his entire right arm becomes paralyzed and he is hospitalized again, this time for surgery. In the course of removing the tumor detected by the angiogram, another, larger tumor is discovered that is not only malignant but inoperable.

When Carl is ready to be discharged from the hospital, his wife decides to care for him at home, hoping to enlist the help of private nurses. But even this first attempt at managing the situation proves difficult: the hospital social worker, whom she sees as opposed to her decision not to institutionalize Carl, only offers her a list of nursing homes, the charitable agencies concerned with cancer care provide no help in securing private nursing, and the physicians seem evasive as to predicting the future course of his illness. After a brief initial period of stabilization, the growth of the tumor is registered in unpredictable seizure activity. It is a difficult time for the Lerners, not just because of the practical problems arising from seizures that can take place at any time and in any place but also because of their helplessness as they watch, with each seizure, a progressive and random deterioration of his condition.[4]

Eventually, the growth of the tumor results in paralysis of Carl's entire right side (confining him to a wheelchair) and the loss of intelligible speech. At this point, he is ready to implement a decision reached in an early phase of his illness—the decision not to allow his life to be prolonged beyond the point where mental or physical impairment makes living intolerable. Having decided to die, he enters the hospital for a medically supervised death, intending to refuse cancer medications as well as life-saving technology. The medical expectation is that the massive steroid withdrawal will lead to coma within seventy-two hours and, then, to death. Although death can to some extent be anticipated, awaited, psychologically prepared for, and even accepted, it is sometimes not so easily programmed. Carl survives for three weeks, not three days, remaining conscious up until the very end.

Not only does Carl's death not conform to the pattern anticipated by his physicians, but the process of dying fits none of the author's own preconceptions. As she observes, "Nothing turned out to be the way literature and myth had told me it would be" (212). For her, the experience of watching her husband die comes to be a process of unlearning, where she must "cut through the myths about dying" and "tear the romantic notions, the lies, out of my head and my feelings" (212). The romantic myth of a shared death here becomes a temptation to be renounced: "All along a dark and terrible urge pulled me toward a total acceptance and sharing of his experience. I cannot say I ever wanted to die with him, rather it was that I felt I was dying with him and must save myself somehow" (264). The title of the book thus takes on an additional plangency: "For the terrible eighteen months of his illness I had struggled to help him to die his own death—in the sense in which Rilke speaks of it—his own death, not mine" (265). The book is written with a wise awareness of what separation by death means, as she realizes that "his own death" implies "her own life."

For both the Lerners, the experience of choosing "one's own death" comes to mean acknowledging the failure of medical predictions, cultural models, and personal expectations. The irony of the book's title is that, originally, it means planning a death that will be one's own but, finally, means dying a death that proves to be one's own precisely by defeating all such plans. Carl Lerner decides to die to avoid the gradual extinction of personality that is so often the result of brain cancer. What thwarts his decision is a deeper element in his own psyche—a commitment to living that does not recognize the rational decision he has made as to the quality of life. The death that turns out to be his is achieved, paradoxically, out of the very failure of his conscious attempt to die.

The discrepancy between the myth of a planned death and the reality of actual dying produces some of the author's most admirably nuanced writing. The entire pathography is informed by her realization that there are multiple truths to contend with in the process of formulation. And in fact, she writes three different endings. The first describes Carl's poignant leave-taking of his son, daughter, and close friends—the benedictory farewells that tradition has led us to expect. The second ending (which she calls "the nightmare version") describes how the death that was so courageously planned keeps eluding him. However, there is a third ending, a philosophic reflection that reconciles both the attempt and the failure to introduce order and meaning into a cancer death; one that does so not so much by dialectically resolving the dissonance of the first two endings as by accepting it. This last version acknowledges that to accept death is also to accept the instinctive need to deny death, even at the very limits of life.

In some sense, this final version serves as the author's formulation—a formulation that distances as it accepts the experience by wisely understanding that the human attempt to make dying heroic or dignified or meaningful may be a response as doomed as it is inevitable. But this is a recognition that the author learns through the course of her experience: it is not the ideological position with which she begins. Indeed, what she records is the failure of the attempt to structure death in ways that seem appropriate for Carl as an individual. It is out of her recognition of this failure that she achieves a kind of learned transcendence—an authenticity of vision that neither affirms nor negates but simply acknowledges.

A Manly Death

Lael Tucker Wertenbaker's *Death of a Man,* as the title suggests, is organized around the paradigm of a death that exemplifies traditional male qualities of courage, virility, and heroism. Published in 1957, twelve years before Kübler-Ross's *On Death and Dying,* this pathography illustrates the regnant cultural attitudes toward hiding and concealing death (both in the United States and on the Continent) that make Kübler-Ross's work so important—and so necessary.[5] Though it is true that today, in the 1990s, a tendency to deny death remains with us, the situation is much improved. The pathography concerns Wertenbaker's husband, a writer by profession, who at age fifty-four discovers he has intestinal cancer. Though it is her narrative, the pathography incorporates sections of a book that he had planned to write about his death. Charles Wertenbaker, when he learns he has cancer, is living in France with his wife and two children. His French doctor urges him to have the tumor removed: he consents to this, deciding to return to New York City for the surgery. At the same time, however, he seriously considers taking his own life by a long and fatal swim out into the ocean, fearing the loss of autonomy and dignity that he assumes will accompany a descent into patienthood: "By then I would be reduced to something less than a man who could swim out to meet his death" (13). He decides against this, his wife reports, one reason being "his feeling that he owed his manhood a test of pain, the bearing of pain, before he died" (16). The remainder of the pathography bears out this devotion to a heroic ideal of manliness.

The author's depiction of the surgeon who is to perform the operation nicely conforms to the organizing myth of "manly death." His entrance is prepared by the appearance of two younger doctors. When the surgeon himself walks into the room, his junior colleagues "snapped to deferent attention"—the military allusion recognizing the surgeon's superiority both in rank and in expertise. In a very long paragraph describing the reasons why one would respect this eminent surgeon, the author first mentions the fact that the surgeon is a very large man, then refers to his self-confidence—which is so great that it is "almost as if he no longer questioned his . . . human liability to error"—and finally, as the crowning achievement, declares that her husband "considered him a man" (41).

Exploratory surgery reveals that the cancer has metastasized to the liver. Nothing is done, in accord with wishes expressed by Wertenbaker and his wife before surgery, and his life expectancy is estimated at three months. Against the advice of his physician, the author tells her husband the truth about his condition. From this point on, medical intervention is rejected, except for palliative measures, and husband and wife appear to be almost conspiratorially engaged in concealing from everyone his fatal prognosis.

Both seem heavily invested in maintaining a mythos of heroism. Though the author denies that they are in any way motivated by such ideas, the way in which she does so betrays the truth she so adamantly denies. Thus, after the breaking of an abscess, for which they have refused medical help, she writes: "There was nothing heroic in our decision to go on dealing with this unforeseen manifestation by the octopus [their words for his cancer] blindly and alone" (103). Her obvious admiration for the way her husband chooses to deal with his approaching death is reflected in comments quoted from other people. So his French doctor is reported as remarking about Wertenbaker, "Madame, un homme magnifique," and as pronouncing later on, when the dying man refuses to be taken to the hospital: "He is the bravest of men. . . . I never in my life expected to meet a man who might face his death this way" (144).

One chapter in the pathography, entitled "The Man They Couldn't Break," is written by Wertenbaker himself, a biography of an idealistic Frenchman who stood up against the Nazis and who was subjected to terrible tortures for doing so. It would seem logical to assume that Wertenbaker saw some analogy between the heroic Frenchman's struggle against the Nazis and his own struggle against cancer or, at least, conceived of this man's heroic suffering as a potential model for his own. His wife at first denies any such analogy: "Wert never for an instant compared his own agonies with the deliberate infliction without alleviation of the greatest possible pain by men on others." Yet, in the very next sentence, her metaphor does suggest that they felt there was a likeness between cancer and the Nazis: "The cancer was an impersonal torturer, although it became for us personified as evil" (141).

Wertenbaker's cancer continues to grow, closing off the left side of the intestines. When he begins to suffer extreme pain, he decides that it is time to end his life. Twice he attempts suicide by injections of morphine; when this fails, he tries to inject an air bubble into a vein. Finally he succeeds in slashing his wrists, unconsciously carrying out the paradigmatic Senecan death that has come down to us in history and literature. A suicide such as this—whether ancient or modern—is meant as a final assertion of control, avoiding a sense of victimization and preventing the gradual diminution and degradation of the personality that are so often the result of prolonged suffering. To prefer an active voluntary death to a passive involuntary one is for the Wertenbakers a strong assertion of manhood.[6]

If the paradigm of heroic death seems to require that the dying man act out his maleness in the arena of death, it also suggests that a complementary role be played by the wife. At one level, *Death of a Man* is all about the attempt of dying husband and surviving wife to integrate terminal illness and death into their relationship. Thus she quotes Wertenbaker in the book he begins to write about his approaching death: "This is [a] search for the essence of perfection in this marriage" (15). And she describes their final night together as they plan his death—he will slash his wrists; she will administer injections of morphine—as characterized by "a kind of final serenity unmatched at any other time." As she injects him with morphine, she cuts her finger on the glass tubes "so that our blood mingled for an instant, symbol of all love" (180).

The idea that death can be shared pervades this pathography; indeed, the book's coauthorship is symbolic of this. This belief in a "shared death" is found in other pathographies as well, where the death of the spouse appears to the survivor as a kind of consummation of their marriage. Thus Martha Weinman Lear, in *Heartsounds,* repeatedly refers to the dress she wears to her husband's funeral as if it were her wedding dress. And in *Last Letter to the Pebble People,* Virginia Hine describes her husband's cancer as "something that was as much a product of our relationship as our children were" and writes that "Aldie even spoke of carrying the cancer in his body for both of us as I had carried our child in my body" (15). In this pathography, the love of husband and wife is seen as triumphing not only over death but also *in* death. So the author writes, in an afterword to her pathography, "I know now that death is truly the fulfillment of love. . . . that death is a necessary part of love. . . . love fulfills itself in death" (158).

In *Death of a Man,* the heroic paradigm of a "manly death" appears to serve an enabling function for both Wertenbaker and his wife. However, this is a myth that can impose heroic demands upon the dying person and family that may make the work of dying more difficult than it need be. It is potentially a dangerous myth in which death becomes something to be "performed"—a summation of the dying man's personality and a validation of his manhood. As Wertenbaker himself remarks, "Dying is the last thing I'll have a chance to do well" (65).

Transcendent Death

A related paradigm appears in *Last Letter to the Pebble People: "Aldie Soars,"* Virginia Hine's enigmatically titled account of the illness and eventual death of her husband, Aldie, from inoperable lung cancer. The quotation in the title—"Aldie Soars"—is the way this man's death is announced to others: it conveys the buoyant sense of victory and transcendence that characterize the conditions of his dying as well as the meaning of his death.

The pathography is organized in two sections—"the Training," with its emphasis on attitude, responsibility, and control, and "the Dying," seen as a process involving stages or graduated "plateaus." It is the second section that concerns us here; the first will be discussed in the following chapter. This second section is organized around the idea of "victorious death," a notion that, after the Hines's long and energetic attempt to reverse the course of Aldie's illness, helps them accept the inevitability of his death. This notion not only functions as a formulation of the death experience but also validates the efforts, the ideologies, and the expectations that went into their attempts to fight the cancer earlier in the narrative, for these are now viewed retrospectively as "training" for death.

Several months before his death, Aldie's condition begins to deteriorate rapidly, as spinal tumors lead to near total paralysis. Despite the fact that his paralysis is considered irreversible, his doctors suggest a combined radiation-chemotherapy program. The author admits that she does not understand the rationale of such a suggestion and then muses: "Maybe life-extension technologies are sometimes a concerned doctor's equivalent of that desperate cry to 'DO something! CHANGE something'"—a compulsion she admits to feeling quite powerfully, at least at first (88). But Aldie easily decides to reject further medical treatment and returns home from the hospital, ready to confront his death.

The kind of death that Aldie prepares for—"victorious death"—seems to be necessarily participatory: it requires a dying person and a group of "survivors," individuals who function both as assistants and as witnesses. Aldie's death is facilitated and observed by some fifteen to twenty family members and close friends, at home, in an ambiance of conviviality and warmth that the author compares to a "house party atmosphere" (104). A death such as this also seems to require a kind of reciprocity on the part of the dying person, who gives some special knowledge to the people who witness his dying. This ritualistic group of the dying person surrounded by an audience is reminiscent of early Christian tracts on the art of dying, where the bystanders help the dying person prepare for death, while *"Moriens"* imparts the wisdom gained from his or her unique and liminal perspective.[7] What Aldie gives to his helper-watchers is a *gnosis* that is psychological and therapeutic rather than spiritual or supernatural. His wife refers to the revelations forced by "the shocking intimacy of a dying person's insight" and comments on "a healing quality in the strange nonverbal communication" that bystanders experience. A death like this, she observes, is for those who attend upon him a "solvent for their angers, their griefs, their jealousies, and tensions" (118, 119, 106).

Virginia and Aldie Hine are lapsed Roman Catholics who "had never been able to find a structure for the spiritual part of ourselves, nor rituals to express feelings and beliefs about the purpose and meaning of life" (82). Hine admits at the beginning of her pathography that "traditional rituals didn't work for us" and dismisses Christmas observances, which occur just days before Aldie's death, with the remark that "none of us were really into

Christmas" (27, 98). Given their distance from traditional religion, it seems at first surprising that an important element in their idea of death is the theme of transcendence. Repeatedly, the process of dying is referred to as a time of transformation (16, 52, 150) or as having a "transcendent quality" (151). The traditional meaning of death-as-transcendence is of course the religious one, where death is the transformation from mortal life and the corruptible body to eternal life and the incorruptible soul. In this pathography, though, the sense of transformation and transcendence survives divorced from any religious meaning.

Religious practices, however, are not so easily separated from their meanings, and the latter return to haunt the pathography in unsettling ways. Respect for the dying person here borders on religious awe: the author refers to "the divinity of Aldie's dying" and compares the discomfort that some feel in Aldie's presence to the uneasiness that people feel "in the presence of a truly holy man" (119, 116). As the process of dying confers upon Aldie himself a kind of sanctity, even his diseased body undergoes a peculiar glorification, so that the odor of cancerous decay is experienced as "sweet and pleasurable" (137). Just such an olfactory miracle was a standard feature in the death of a great many Roman Catholic saints. If the author here seems unaware of the link between this particular perception and religious convention, she is fully conscious of the connection when she describes an incident where Aldie moves his hands towards her "as if to give me something very precious," and she is reminded of "receiving the wafer at the communion rail all those years ago when we still went to church" (133). As though to emphasize the presence of a powerful religious mythos, looking at this dying man's distorted body Hine sees "a Christ-likeness . . . the beauty of Christ shrouding him like an aura" and a friend determines to "bring her camera the next day to get a picture of Christ" (136–37).

The language of strained transcendence in which Aldie is described here, along with the extravagant images of Christ or a dying saint, suggests the extent to which all the actors in this drama are trying hard to make the myth of the transcendent death work for them. In this pathography of a nontraditional couple who see their love for each other as the purpose and end of their lives, and who perceive their "flow-through" house, open to kin and nonkin, as a substitute for a spiritual structure (82), Roman Catholic images and themes suggest the emotional ambiance though not the doctrinal meaning of Christianity. The ritual celebration of Mass with its communion wafer, the sweet odor of a dying saint, the redemptive qualities of a Christ-like death, and the image of the crucified Christ, so powerful to anyone with a Roman Catholic childhood—all these return as fragments of a religion divorced from their meaning. Whether or not they are divorced from their function as offering consolation is a question of interpretation.

One might argue that this pathography chronicles the successful liberation of those aspects of religion that are truly consoling from their source in meaningless dogma and blind faith. But the reader cannot fail to come away from this book disturbed. At the very least, the work of dying seems to have been made more arduous by the demand that it be a performance—and a performance imbued with the myth of sacred death—"dying well." The author writes that Aldie, on the morning of his death, talks with presences he calls Death and Love, affirming his readiness to die. Given the script of a "transcendent death" that dictates the meaning and the manner of this man's dying, one wonders if a conversation with abstractions is an adequate substitute for the ritual prayers to a higher power that traditionally accompanied the art of "dying well."

Easy Death

Each of the pathographies discussed so far concerns the death of a spouse. As one might expect, pathographies written about the death of an elderly parent are somewhat different. Because the dying parent is so often represented as denying death, there is no attempt at heroism, no attempt to individualize or personalize death, and no attempt to find meaning in the experience on the part of the dying person. The paradigm for these pathographies is that of "easy death." This paradigm has an immediate source in the nineteenth century with the Victorian concern to euphemize death. People did not die then; they "passed away," a phrase still in use in some circles today (and reflected in the contemporary medical term "expired"). The notion of death implied in this euphemism is the culmination of a gradual process of diminishing day by day—an image perfectly epitomized in the famous photograph called "Fading Away" by Julia Cameron. In the novels of Charles Dickens, the deaths of children, especially, were sentimentalized in this way: one thinks of the pathos in the death of "little Nell" in *The Old Curiosity Shop*. At a time when the mortality rate for children was extremely high, the need for such comforting euphemisms was imperative.[8] Today, though, the death of an elderly parent has replaced the death of a child as an ordeal central to many of us, and it is euphemized getting well" (77). At one point, de Beauvoir quotes the concern of a friend of her mother's: "Since she is in such a state of anxiety, she must surely want the comforts of religion." To this the daughter replies—her deception here colluding with her mother's denial—"What she wants just now is to be helped to make a good recovery" (90).

"Maman" had been a pious Roman Catholic all her life, and de Beauvoir expresses surprise that her religion seems to mean so little to her during her last days: she never asks for a priest, repeatedly refuses Communion, and never once uses the missal, crucifix, and rosary brought to her in the hospital. De Beauvoir's explanation for this seems evasive: she projects her own intellectual attitude on her mother, observing that "Maman loved life as I love it and in the face of death she had the same feeling of rebellion that I have" (91). The real explanation, of course, is the deception visited on this dying woman by everyone around her: why should she turn to the consolations of religion if she is convinced that she is recovering from peritonitis?

Key to the myth of easy death is the avoidance of suffering. "In this race between pain and death," writes de Beauvoir, "we most earnestly hoped that death would come first" (75). This pathography is constructed out of the tension between the author's own intense fear of death, which is expressed in consenting to operations that prolong her mother's suffering as well as her life, and her wish that her mother die painlessly and easily. As in other pathographies about a dying parent, the author is bitter about the mechanical insistence on medical intervention and the marked lack of compassion that characterize her mother's primary physician. For this doctor, who is "infatuated with technique," her mother is "the subject of an interesting experiment and not a person" (52).

When her mother finally dies, de Beauvoir is not present. The story is told through the responses of her sister, who breaks down at the horror of the final moment of death. She describes her mother in the last vestiges of consciousness: "Her mouth opened, her eyes stared wide, huge in that wasted, ravaged face: with a spasm she entered into coma." Betrayed by the doctors' promise that her mother "would go out like a candle," the sister sobs, "it wasn't like that, it wasn't like that at all." In response, the nurse in attendance tries to comfort her: "But, Madame . . . I assure you it was a very easy death" (88). The formula that gives the book its title is of course an ironic one. The author seems obsessed throughout the pathography with the sight of her mother's mutilated and tormented body, which, even

in a similar way: "an easy death" replaces the "fading away" of Vict
thanatology.

Simone de Beauvoir's pathography is a powerful and moving des
tion of the final illness and death of her elderly mother and her own
tempts to do what seems best for her. A major twentieth-century wi
for whom death and the absurd are central topics, this famous French l
wing intellectual, early feminist, and lifelong companion of Jean-P.
Sartre must here find a balance between her philosophic theories abc
death and her own actual feelings, thoughts, and actions as she confror
the reality of her mother's dying. Her first response to the idea that h
mother might die is dispassionate: "After all, she was of an age to die" (12
But in witnessing, day by day and hour by hour, the gradual deterioration
of her mother's condition, she comes to see her simplistic formulae abou
death as untrue to the horror of its reality and the depth of her own feeling.

The narrative begins when de Beauvoir is called home to be with her
mother, who has been hospitalized after a fall. When X-rays reveal the presence of a tumor blocking the small intestine, her doctors advise surgery.
"Maman" is told neither of the probable cancer nor even of the impending operation. Though a nurse warns the author, "Don't let her be oper-
ated on!" she nonetheless gives permission for the surgery, but not without
misgivings (28). The nurse's warning returns like a refrain to haunt her later
on as she watches her mother slowly die. She blames herself for not
preventing this operation but feels that she had been overwhelmed by
the medical machine: "One is caught up in the wheels and dragged
along, powerless in the face of specialists' diagnoses, their forecasts, their
decisions" (57).

Remarking that her mother had always feared cancer and expected to
die from it, de Beauvoir concurs with the physicians' decision not to inform her that she has cancer.[9] Accordingly, "Maman" is told that she suffers from peritonitis. Though de Beauvoir writes of this as an act of
"betrayal" resulting in loneliness on the part of the sick woman and re-
morse on the part of her family, she never reverses the decision and never
tells her mother the truth. She does not express regret for this deception,
as she did about permitting the operation, but the narrative itself betrays
her ambivalence as she keeps returning to the futility of her mother's desperate attempts to get well: "She rested and dreamed," the author observes,
"infinitely far removed from her rotting flesh, her ears filled with the sound
of our lies; her whole person was concentrated upon one passionate hope—

before she dies, is literally rotting away. Near the end her eyes appear huge in her wasted face, her smile is "the macabre grin of a skeleton," her body is swollen and blue from edema, the surgical wound in her abdomen is open and festering, and her emaciated thighs and hips are covered with bedsores. She requires massive doses of morphine to alleviate her pain. And, despite all this, up until the very end Madame de Beauvoir apparently doesn't even know she is dying. The "easy death" here may extend not only to the awful details of her mother's dying but also to the consolation intended by the deceit of those who love and tend her.

De Beauvoir's final understanding appears to glance away from the terrible image of a grotesque and mutilated body and the conspiracy of deceit surrounding her mother's death. She concludes on a philosophic note with the assertion that "there is no such thing as a natural death" and that death, for each of us, is an accident and, even if we consent to it, an "unjustifiable violation." One wonders if the irony of this book's title, *A Very Easy Death* (or, in the French, *Une Mort Très Douce*), does not convey a more accurate sense of this author's ambiguous and troubled formulation than do these simplistic existentialist pronouncements about death as *"le scandale,"* a meaningless and irrational evil.

One might counter that de Beauvoir's book, first published in France in 1964, was written before recent important changes in medical ethics, such as truth-telling and informed consent, had come about; moreover, one could argue that French culture remains to this day more paternalistic in its medical ethics, especially concerning truthfulness about cancer. But Le Anne Schreiber's *Midstream,* published in the United States in 1990, also a pathography about a mother's death from cancer, shares with de Beauvoir's narrative the same pervasive attitude of denial and the same preoccupation with alleviation or elimination of pain—two components of the paradigm of easy death. Despite the fact that Schreiber, her physician-brother, and her mother's doctors are all well aware of the statistical probability that this woman with pancreatic cancer will not live very long, her cancer is treated aggressively with surgery and radiation. The result is the same as in the de Beauvoir pathography: the elderly patient dutifully does everything possible "to get better," and yet everyone around her knows at some level that this is not going to happen—a knowledge they themselves proceed to deny in various ways.

Throughout Schreiber's pathography, the sick woman refuses to accept the idea that she might not recover from her illness. Radically weakened either by the disease or by the drugs used to treat it, unable to walk without help, and with her weight steadily decreasing, she refuses to use the wheelchair her daughter has bought for her and rejects all but the most basic assistance in nursing care, insisting that "until I'm on my feet again, the less intrusion from the outside world the better" (205). Little more than a week before she dies, she asks to be taken to the hospital, again denying that her condition might be anything but temporary: "Maybe they can make me well, find out what's wrong with my legs; I know it isn't cancer" (250). The day before her death she asks the priest who now visits her daily with communion if she is "going to be all right" (272). Ironically, he answers in the affirmative, thinking she is asking about the condition of her soul.

The author attributes her mother's denial in part to temperament and in part "because the doctors at the medical center continually misled her" (198). Specifically, she is referring to her mother's oncologist, who, when she visits him with a complaint of back pain, is reported as announcing: "Mrs. Schreiber, there is nothing more we can do for you. You are cured. You are no longer a cancer patient" (120). The author finds the mention of cure outrageous, as does her physician-brother. Most probably, Schreiber intends us to see this oncologist not as exhibiting denial but simply lying in order to rid himself of a patient who is no longer a candidate for aggressive medical treatment. His remarks are further motivated, the author suspects, by the wish "to wash his hands of the messy problem of pain" (120).

A pernicious form of medical denial is the way the physicians in this pathography actually do deal with this woman's pain, which is frequently demoted to the euphemism "discomfort," discounted as unimportant, or seen as a condition for which she must seek help elsewhere. These doctors, the author remarks with bitterness, "are specialists trained to intervene at moments of crisis, to cut, to radiate, to alter chemistry," a training that does not prepare them "for sustained care of the human being who continues to feel the effects of the doctors' knives and beams and chemicals" (138). In one memorable instance, the medical team decides to control Mrs. Schreiber's pain with a nerve block—an elaborate and potentially dangerous procedure that fails totally. Frustrated and desperate, she consults a Chinese doctor skilled in acupuncture who uses a TENS machine (transcutaneous electrical nerve stimulator) for her pain, with immediate and drastic positive results. What seems most troubling about this episode is that the anesthesiologist who performs the nerve block knows about this simple method for pain relief, considers it "very effective," and yet never offers it as a therapeutic option (158).

All the characters in *Midstream* are affected by the denial that pervades this woman's illness. Thus, at one point, Schreiber herself is convinced that her mother's general deterioration, especially her loss of muscle tone in the calf and her resulting inability to walk, is caused by the prednisone and Elavil she has been given and not by any recurrence or spread of the cancer. The author's brother debunks this theory as "denial." However, not long after, this same doctor-brother also comes up with an alternate explanation for his mother's physical deterioration, theorizing that her decline may be caused not by cancer but by hypothyroidism (she had been given an oral dose of radioactive iodine for hyperthyroidism some twenty years ago). Even the hospice nurse attending Mrs. Schreiber becomes "infected" with denial, and various procedures are ordered to determine thyroid levels. But test results rule out both these theories as clinical possibilities.

Denial is a pathological syndrome here, accompanying and even rivaling Mrs. Schreiber's pancreatic cancer as the book's thematic center. Repeatedly, the author describes denial in medical metaphors: "Maybe denial is catching, and we've infected her [the hospice nurse]" or "I was succumbing to another bout of denial" or "Dad caught a full-blown case of denial from Mom" (226, 219, 251). The pervasive "disease" of denial even survives Mrs. Schreiber's death. Thus, at his wife's wake, Mr. Schreiber assures the many mourners and visitors that his wife did not suffer a great deal in her last few months. Indeed, the made-up corpse in the open casket seems to verify this story: mourners who had not seen Mrs. Schreiber in her last months of life "see her as if she had been mysteriously struck down in the pink of good health" (283). The author is appalled by all this. She observes, "I thought death would end denial, but it just ushers in a new phase of it. First we deny that death is coming, and then, when it's arrived, we pretend the coming was peaceful" (285).

Denial in both de Beauvoir's and Schreiber's pathographies makes difficult the necessary choices between surgical intervention that would prolong life and the withholding of treatment that would spare a terminal patient additional pain. The notion of "easy death" is the mythic solution to the burden of impossible choices like these. Given the reality of pain and our prevailing cultural ethos of denial, perhaps the paradigm of an easy death is the best we can do. It is true that it spares an elderly person the need to be heroic, or to undergo spiritual calisthenics in preparation for death, or to perform in some way for an audience of onlookers—models for dying exhibited in pathographies discussed earlier in this chapter. But its limitations are manifold. To die with no comprehension of what is happening diminishes what is human about us, creates a systematic framework of deceit, and contributes to a profound loneliness on the part of both the dying and the survivors.

At some level, denial may well be an instinctive response to death for all of us; Kübler-Ross sees it as our initial reaction. There does indeed seem to be a kind of "life wish," some force that makes us assert life even at the edge of death. The ability of an elderly person with a terminal illness to deny the imminence of death seems a special instance of this life force—a force that often asserts itself in inverse proportion to the time remaining. Given this almost biological tenacity to hold onto life the closer one actually gets to death, our lack of any art of dying that would help the elderly who are terminally ill in accepting death does everyone a great disservice. The doctor who practices an ethic of denial by mechanically insisting on prolongation of life can in fact do a good deal of harm, in paradoxical violation of the Hippocratic oath. And the individual who deceives an elderly parent as to diagnosis or prognosis may be sparing him or her the terror of imminent death, but the result is that the parent is confused as to why the recovery that is anticipated does not take place, denied the support and consolation of loved ones, and deprived of an opportunity to come to terms with death.

If our cultural habit of denying death is so disastrous for all concerned—and I do believe it is—then we would expect a pathography where death is accepted to offer a more beneficial approach to the death of a parent. Philip Roth's *Patrimony* seems just such a pathography, a book that is partly an encomium on Herman Roth and partly the story of this man's gradual decline into death. Early in the narrative, Roth discovers that his eighty-six-year-old father has a massive brain tumor. Though he finds it difficult to tell him—a difficulty given narrative form in the fact that some fifty pages elapse between his receiving the bad news and telling it to his father—he does so, and with great tact. It is the *son*, not the father, who agonizes over what should be done, observing that "[I was] unconvinced that there was any reward commensurate with the risks involved in surgery, yet conscious that if nothing was done, *in a relatively short time* his condition could deteriorate horribly" (145). That Herman Roth himself can accept death is made clear when he refuses to undergo the drastic but potentially life-extending surgery recommended by the several neurosurgeons he consults. He has little difficulty in making a decision when the time comes. His wry refusal of further surgery is in striking contrast to the denial characteristic of the de Beauvoir and Schreiber pathographies: "Well, Doctor," he remarks, "I've got a lot of people waiting for me on the other side" (164).

There are several aspects of this pathography that render it different from others, and some elements that seem deeply troubling. At first glance, *Patrimony* is remarkable for its relative lack of the self-scrutiny and ambivalence so common to most pathographies about a dying parent. Here we do not find feelings of anger and resentment, fantasies of denial, or "selfish" attempts to cling to one's own life. Instead, we sense self-congratulation— or perhaps justification—as Roth plays the role of the dutiful son with admirable if uninflected scrupulosity. *Patrimony* is a well-crafted and even moving book, but—partly as a result of this simplified self-characterization—it does not seem to be a "psychological" book. And this is surprising, given the fact that Roth is also the author of a book that is virtually a literary exercise in psychoanalysis—*Portnoy's Complaint.*

Patrimony, however, is more complicated than at first it might appear. Given the peculiar absence here of the kind of naive self-reflection so typical of pathography, it is possible to read *Patrimony*—with the important exception of the dream reported at the very end—as wishful fantasy. Throughout the narrative, Roth feels and acts as we all *ought* to during this most difficult rite of passage. But this exaggerated emphasis on doing "the right thing" paradoxically results in passages that feel wrong—passages that signal an undoing of the book's apparent self-justification. The first such passage is Roth's discussion of some love letters that his father, recently widowed, had sent to a woman in whom he was romantically interested. As Roth describes these letters, and even quotes from them, one wonders at the son's audacity in reading them at all and the author's further transgression in making public something so private. Another such entry is Roth's description of his father in the bath. As he bathes the old man he stares fixedly at his penis, remarking on its size, comparing it to his own, reflecting on the pleasure it must have given to both father and mother, and reminding himself "to fix it in my memory for when he was dead" (177).[10]

In these two episodes Roth violates, first symbolically and then literally, the Old Testament taboo against "uncovering thy father's nakedness." That he feels he has done so is confirmed by the dream that concludes the pathography, a nightmare in which his father returns "in a hooded white shroud" to reproach his son because he "had dressed him for eternity in the wrong clothes" (237). On the literal level, the dream refers to Roth's decision to bury his father in a tallis, "the shroud of our ancestors," rather than a business suit. This is very much an idealization: Herman Roth, the New Jersey businessman, becomes Herman Roth, the Jewish patriarch. On a deeper level (and this is clearly Roth's interpretation), the dream refers to the pathography itself, "which, in keeping with the unseemliness of my profession, I had been writing all the while he was ill and dying" (237). Not only, then, do some of the book's entries encroach on his father's privacy, but the entire pathography can be seen as an exercise in exploitation—the professional writer finding material for his next book in his father's final illness and death. Though the pathography pays tribute to Herman Roth— "Philip Roth's most irrepressible and irresistible hero yet," according to the book jacket—it also *uses* him, and the dream is evidence that Roth is aware of this fact.

This concluding dream rescues the narrative that precedes it from being a kind of pathographical Emily Post on the death of a parent. It highlights, in retrospect, too-personal episodes like those discussed above and prevents the reader from seeing the pathography as idealizing Roth's role in caring for his dying father. Indeed, the title suggests that this is Roth's own interpretation. For the "patrimony" that Herman Roth gives his son is "not the money," which he has given to his other son, "not the tefillin," ritual artifacts of Orthodox Judaism that he has abandoned in a locker at the local YMCA, and "not the shaving mug" handed down from his own father, "but the shit," which the author cleans up after his father lost control of his bowels (176). The realization comes to him as a kind of epiphany: "So *that* was the patrimony. And not because cleaning it up was symbolic of something else but because it wasn't, because it was nothing less or more than the lived reality that it was" (176).

The key to this pathography is the book's title, *Patrimony,* with its mythic meaning of heritage, birthright, and inheritance, and its personal meaning, for Roth, of "lived reality" itself—with all its obligations, its ordinariness, and its attention to bodily functions. Read in this way, the pathography is much more than simply a sentimental, self-indulgent, and unreflective eulogy of a dying parent. The mythic version of how to negotiate the death of a parent is rendered as realistic fiction—"a true story," to quote the paradoxical and clichéd subtitle of the pathography—whereas the other version, the "lived reality," appears as a symbolic nightmare re-constituted in Roth's interpretation. What we are left with is an irrevocable split between the myth, which is recorded as narrative, and the reality, which reveals itself in the interstices of the story.

It is true that Roth's pathography, unlike those of de Beauvoir and Schreiber, is free from the myth of an easy death and devoid of the habit of denial that seems to accompany this myth. However, the attitude of acceptance that distinguishes this pathography from others seems allied to an idealization of both father and son that may be overcompensatory. *Patrimony* beautifully delineates the mythic expectations of how one ought to act when confronting the death of a parent—and then explodes them.

"Facing" Death

Peter Noll's *In the Face of Death,* a book originally published in Switzerland in 1984 and translated into English in 1989, is an unusual pathography about death—unusual because, with the exception of the final chapter, it is written by the dying person himself. As the title suggests, this pathography is the very reverse of the pattern of "easy death." Neither denial nor the avoidance of pain are primary objectives here: Noll's "Socratic calm would indulge anything except consolation," maintains the friend who gives his funeral oration (249). *In the Face of Death* is a useful conclusion to this chapter on pathographies about dying because it subsumes most of the other mythic patterns we have been observing: the manner in which Noll confronts dying is very much one of his own choosing, it conforms to philosophic and heroic models, and it even resonates with certain beliefs central to the Christian faith.

Noll is a Swiss professor of criminal law, divorced, with two grown daughters. He is also an accomplished writer on a variety of topics ranging from jurisprudence to philosophy and religion. His medical story begins with pain in the left kidney. The urologist diagnoses cancer of the bladder, recommending a bladder resection that may save his life but will leave him impotent and able to urinate only by means of an artificial opening into a plastic bag attached to his abdomen. Noll immediately decides against such surgery even before his doctor finishes speaking, determined not to lose his freedom and self-respect by "get[ting] caught in the surgical-urological-radiological machine" (5). Though he realizes that his decision not to pursue treatment denies him any chance of survival, he is content with this choice, feeling that he is "choos[ing] metastasis" rather than a "technological prolongation of death" (3). One senses a strong life-affirming element in Noll's decision to refuse treatment, though this expresses itself not in the wish to prolong life but in the desire to preserve a certain quality of life. This is evident in the careful way in which he describes landscape and weather, in the pleasure he takes in physical activities like skiing, in his apparent enjoyment of an active sexual life, and in the gusto and delight with which he eats and drinks. For Noll, a medical death, with "each of one's body's orifices . . . hooked up to a tube," is to be avoided at all costs: "The urge to survive must never be allowed to become so absolutely over-powering that one submits to all of these indignities. The will to live must oppose it" (20).

Noll has an advantage over most patients in that he has a brother who is a doctor, an "insider" who can translate the reports of the radiologist and urologist, evaluate the medical advice he has been given about bladder resection, and interpret the statistical evidence tendered in support of it. This brother's role in the decisions recorded in the pathography is a major one. Thus, Noll can remark that while his physicians were certainly candid with him, they were "not completely honest" about the surgical procedure they recommended—one that really offered only a thirty-percent chance of survival, according to his doctor-brother, not the fifty-percent figure given him by his urologist—and this for only a period of five years. The troubling implication is that doctors often do not tell patients the truth, especially if they sense that a patient is skeptical about treatment, as Noll clearly is; and that if they did, more people might question the wisdom of assenting to procedures that tend only to prolong life, often at the price of great physical and psychological pain. The conclusion Noll draws is that his doctors are motivated in everything they say and do by the principle of acting to preserve life. Moreover, he sees the unqualified determination to prolong life as characteristic not just of his own doctors but of the profession itself: "The compulsion to preserve life at any price—only in the medical profession do we encounter it palpably and systematically" (139).

The clarity and certainty that characterize Noll's decision to reject medical intervention illustrate the benefits of an attitude that does not deny death, in marked contrast to the pathographies discussed above as examples of "easy death." His "negative" decision to reject medical intervention is accompanied by a positive motive—to use the time remaining to prepare for death and look it "squarely in the face" (19). That his approach should seem so radical to us, and that his book should be nearly unique among pathographies about dying, is a measure of how divorced we are from such an approach. What he is describing (and what his book documents) is an attitude toward death consistent in many ways with the *ars moriendi* tradition of older, more religious cultures. Noll is of course the *Moriens* and his readers the bystanders, who, if they cannot assist him during his dying, benefit from the perceptions and reflections that make up his pathography. Noll describes how he makes his will, plans his memorial service, and even writes his own funeral sermon. Repeatedly he speculates on the problem of an afterlife. Pondering the meaning of death, he gives to his readers a sense of life perceived from the unique perspective of the dying.

If Noll's pathography reminds one of an *ars moriendi* handbook, it also looks back to the philosophic traditions of Socrates and the Stoics in Noll's discussions of suicide, in his determination not to sacrifice his dignity and freedom by submitting to institutional control (whether medical or political), and in the fact that so much of the texture of this book is conversation with friends—a modern version of the philosophic circle. Noll's decision to refuse treatment—by example a rebuke to "the medical machine"—is in a way analogous to Socrates' refusal to bow to the authority of the new Athenian democracy. Socrates sees his own death as a better alternative to living under the political tyranny of his day; Noll welcomes the opportunity "to look death squarely in the face" as an improvement over "the medical-technical death-ritual" (19, 16).

In the Face of Death is in many ways an impressive document. It is much more than a medical memoir: it blends Noll's reflections on such themes as politics, religion, theology, law, and, of course, pain and death, with brief entries on the status of his illness. It is a journal written, he says, "to give meaning to my dying and death, a meaning also for others in the same situation" (210). Noll is in the tradition of the great philosophers of the West in associating proximity to death with the opportunity of becoming wise. His thoughts on dying are in the same vein as those of Seneca and Montaigne—in fact, he quotes Montaigne in a passage advocating the benefits of a preoccupation with death during one's life, the essential freedom in the act of dying, and the nobility in fully accepting one's death (32–33). But the meaning Noll gropes for is one paradoxically achieved out of the impossibility of meditating on death. Death, he remarks, is nothingness, total senselessness, the *totaliter aliter*. What is called for in confronting and accepting one's own dying is a concern with life, "life in the face of death, life viewed from the perspective of death" (62).

Noll feels that the imminence of his death offers him a valuable perspective on life, and this view of life *sub specie mortalitatis* is what he offers to the readers of his pathography. His decision to reject medical intervention is unsettling for many friends and acquaintances and downright threatening for some of the doctors he encounters: he sees their discomfort as a measure of our cultural investment in denying death and the result of being suddenly "challenged to confront dying and death as a part of life" (45). Noll calls for a reform of funeral rituals, convinced that they ought "to present death clearly and to nurture the thought of death" rather than "suppress the reality of dying and death," as they now do. Moreover, our funerary rites, he remarks, ought "to be critical of the medical-technical death-ritual," counterbalancing the medical denial of death by helping us accept death and prepare ourselves for it (15–16).

The organizing myth here is not that of "holy dying," and the model is certainly not one of a transcendent death. But the Christian idea of the resurrection does find its way into this narrative, though it does so obliquely. It achieves realization in the music Noll selects for his memorial service—Bach's B-Minor Mass, with its powerful choral rendition of the crucifixion in *"sepultus est"* and the "triumphal victory over death" in the next section, the *"Et resurrexit."* Though he clearly states that he does not believe in the orthodox Christian notion of resurrection, yet Noll also admits that this music, with its resounding affirmation of "a triumph over death," is linked to the reason that he does not fear dying. Without compromising his intellectual integrity, Noll permits those intimations of reality that are nonlogical, nonrational, and nonverbal to affect his total understanding of the experience of death. That he can feel overwhelmed by "the idea of an eternal kingdom of God, *whether I experience it or not"* [48; italics mine], is simultaneously a disavowal of any personal belief in an afterlife and at the same time a profound statement of faith.

The final chapter of this pathography, written by Noll's daughter after her father's death, offers in its tone, intent, and style a very different perspective on Noll's project of facing death. Throughout the last month or so of his illness, Noll tries to balance the need to remain fully conscious, which he must do if he is truly to face his own death, with the ever-increasing problem of pain. He readily takes morphine when the pain becomes unendurable but is disconcerted when, increasingly, the amount of morphine needed causes confusion and disorientation. His daughter tells how Noll becomes lost and apparently spends several days, delirious, in a nearby park after taking a large dose of morphine. When she finds him, he is hallucinating—"looking for young, talented painters," as he remarks—and remains so for several days. When he recovers, he feels such shame at his loss of control that he decides to stop using morphine entirely—a decision he stands by until his death a week or so later. Throughout this time he appears to be in great agony. His daughter moves in with him near the end, even sleeping on the bed with him during his last days, until he dies in her arms.

Early in his pathography, Noll observes that pain is meaningful for such as "Jesus and the martyrs [who] were suffering *for something.*" He determines that "to bear pain, to endure it, proves the superiority of the spirit over life." However, for the terminal cancer patient, he goes on to observe, to endure willingly unendurable pain is pointless: "Here all attempts to see any deeper meaning must stop, and the only thing left is morphine" (32). Given these earlier thoughts, his decision near the end of his life to refuse morphine because "death assumes a higher quality when it is more conscious" (155) seems all the more remarkable.

Noll's decision to forego morphine so that he can remain lucid—a decision whose consequence is that he dies in considerable pain—suggests a philosophic or even a heroic death. For the daughter who witnesses his suffering, the impression is rather different. Trying to comfort him, she thinks of the crucified Christ: "It occurred to me that somebody else had endured this agony, and I talked to him about Jesus on the cross." Her subsequent remark, "Even the Son of God despaired in the face of death" is an ironic reflection on the implicit heroism of the book's title. When Noll dies, in great pain, in her arms, she thinks to herself: "My God, how can you let anybody suffer like this!" (247).

Rebekka Noll's final chapter shows the same unflinching candor that makes her father's pathography so admirable, and for this very reason, it forces the reader to reexamine the premises on which Noll acts. Is the consciousness he so prizes worth the pain he suffers? But if the only alternative is drug-induced coma or delusion, could we wish that for him—or for ourselves?

Of all the pathographies that deal with dying, I find Noll's the most impressive, not because it provides a model for death in our time but, in part, because it does not. Noll dies in the way he freely, spontaneously, and knowingly chooses: it is, we feel, the "right death" for him. But we cannot go on to assert that it would be the right death for others. Not everyone could accept such appalling pain or value so highly the benefits of philosophical reflection. One lesson to be drawn from Noll's pathography—a pathography that seems in many ways so close to a modern *ars moriendi*—is that perhaps there can be no art of dying, which is by nature a universalizing construct, in a culture that values individuality and emphasizes pluralism. One might even go so far as to assert that the absence of such a paradigm is really a benefit to us, since mythic expectations of the "right death" or the "good death" or an "easy death" can, as we have seen, be cruelly inaccurate.

Indeed, what may be most problematic is not the absence of a viable, contemporary *ars moriendi,* but the frantic and uncritical way in which we seem to be creating individual versions of how to die. Perhaps one reason why the work of dying seems so difficult today is that the individual is expected not only to face his or her death—in itself a task arduous enough—but also to create a way of dying out of the fragments of ideologies and religious sentiments that our culture provides us. Though this may be inevitable in the modern world, it is a situation that can be problematic for many of us. Perhaps the pathographical formulations discussed above, in their emphases on structuring, sharing, planning, or even "experiencing" death, tend to lose sight of death as, simply, the end of life. And if death is simply the end of life, then it becomes a mystery to be confronted, not an experience that can be possessed by or assimilated into the personality. Perhaps what is needed is the realization, as Gerda Lerner puts it, that death may well be simply the "other side of life" (269)—random, inevitable, and unknowable.

CHAPTER FIVE

✴

Healthy-Mindedness: Myth as Medicine

Pathographies in recent years show a dramatic increase in the frequency with which patients turn to alternative medicine—a term for therapies and approaches that often have little in common except for the fact that they are *not* a part of the traditional biomedical model. They include ancient treatment modalities of other cultures as well as "pop" treatments spawned by the New Age movement, therapies with scientific documentation of their effectiveness and therapies that seem clearly the product of greed and charlatanism, treatments that strike one as eminently commonsensical and treatments that seem naive or fanciful. To name but a few, alternative therapies include acupuncture and shiatsu, Reiki, macrobiotics, Ayurveda and polarity therapy, healing crystals and other Native American practices, homeopathy, naturopathy, anthroposophical medicine, Issels' Whole-Body Therapy, Livingston Therapy, Nieper's eumetabolic therapy, Laetrile, psychosynthesis, Hoxsey Therapy and the Bach Flower Remedies, Gerson therapy and other detoxification regimens, Rolfing and Aston-Patterning, the many schools of image-therapy and the many techniques of meditation, iridology, reflexology and myotherapy, past life therapy, psychic healing, and the cultivation of lucid dreaming. I omit from this list any reference to holistic medicine, though it is often used as a synonym for alternative medicine, because the term has such varied meanings.[1]

For most pathographers, alternative medicine is a reactive way of thinking and feeling—a response to perceived inadequacies in the current biomedical model. Though, strictly speaking, many current alternative modalities predate biomedicine (some by thousands of years), nonetheless most pathographers rediscover and turn to them in disillusionment, frustration, or anger at orthodox medicine. Seen from this perspective—with biomedicine at the center—the many forms of alternative medicine are characterized by what orthodox medicine is not. If the model of patient-hood in biomedicine is one of passivity, in alternative medicine the model is one of agency—the patient is expected to be a fully involved participant in his or her own therapy. If in biomedicine specific treatments are veri-fied by statistical evidence, in alternative medicine verification is arrived at by anecdotal evidence—the fact that a given therapy has worked for some people. In biomedicine, it is the disease that often seems to be the focus; in alternative medicine, the individual with the disease. Biomedicine is al-lied with technology; alternative medicine is associated with natural agents and processes. There seems to be no single center to the actual practices associated with alternative medicine: their configurations are multiple, re-acting to various aspects of the biomedical model. Health care today is like a jigsaw puzzle with biomedicine at the center and the various alternative therapies organized around it, the shape of each determined by the con-tours of its antagonist.[2]

The striking increase over the last ten years in pathographies describ-ing alternative medical therapies may reflect increased use of such mo-dalities by the general population. Moreover, it is possible that such pathographies, in their capacity to serve as models, may themselves influ-ence the ease and frequency with which patients turn to these methods. It is well to remember that for every pathography in print documenting the helpfulness of visualization exercises, or Laetrile, or herbal remedies, there are thousands of individual readers. The extent to which sick persons in America today will seek out alternative modes of treatment should be trou-bling to the medical establishment because it is evidence not just of a dis-satisfaction with particular physicians but also of a lack of confidence in the methods and principles of biomedical science itself. Health care today has become a commodity, and orthodox medicine, despite its continuing legal and economic hegemony in the United States, no longer has a mo-nopoly over it. Increasingly, patients are unwilling to tolerate a kind of medical treatment that, however technologically sophisticated, casts them into the role of passive and depersonalized recipient; increasingly, they are reluctant to submit to therapies that are painful, invasive, and unlikely to result in cure. More and more, ill people are not content to settle for dis-ease management: instead, they want to be healed.

But the turn to alternative medicine is motivated by something deeper than dissatisfaction with orthodox medicine. As one might expect, there is a mythic component in the allure of many kinds of alternative medical therapies—a constellation of attitudes and beliefs that might be called *healthy-mindedness*. This is my subject here: not alternative medicine as such, but healthy-mindedness—a mythos frequently (though not always) invoked in the use of alternative therapies.[3] The term itself is one I have borrowed from the great American psychologist and philosopher, William James. At the turn of the century, in his *Varieties of Religious Experience*, James commented on a current of thinking "which has recently poured over America and seems to be gathering force every day" (87). He was referring to such movements as faith healing and Christian Science, a growing interest in parapsychology, and a marked detachment from orthodox Christianity. James associated these movements with a stance toward life that he called "the religion of healthy-mindedness"—an attitude characterized by the sense that nature is inherently and absolutely good, the relegation of evil and sin to the status of illusory constructs, a belief in the "conquering efficacy" of the positive emotions, and a relentless optimism— a stance that he contrasted to that of the "sick soul" (76–139).[4] Those blessed with healthy-mindedness live in a one-dimensional universe governed by a beneficent Nature, where all one need do to "live right" is to love others, be happy, and exercise one's mind in the pursuit of optimistic thoughts. For the sick soul, on the contrary, the felt presence of fear, guilt, and despair and the intrusion of evil in the world render a "healthy-minded" attitude not only impossible to maintain but a flagrant distortion of reality.

The religious attitudes that James detected a century ago have been reinforced in our own time by the increased interest in all forms of Eastern religious thought and practice and in the spiritualism of the New Age movement.[5] But until very recently, the medical theories and practices that reflect such attitudes have been eclipsed by the twentieth-century hegemony of biomedicine, institutionalized in the American Medical Association. Politically and economically, the long contest between homeopaths and their victorious allopathic rivals ended shortly after the appearance of the Flexner report in 1910, when state licensing required an AMA approved medical school. The appearance of sulfa drugs in the 1930s, making possible the cure of bacterial pneumonia, meningitis, and gonorrhea, further legitimized the biomedical approach, as did the discovery of penicillin and other antibiotics in the 1940s. It seemed apparent that scientific research was the key to better medical treatment. While the alliance between science and medicine was strengthened, the link between the medical and the humanistic became ever more tenuous. Medicine's primary concern shifted away from the welfare of the individual patient and toward the diagnosis and treatment of disease.

More recently, biomedicine has slipped from its brief position of uncontested authority in all aspects of health care. The reasons are multiple: pressures of government programs such as Medicaid and Medicare, intervention by insurance companies, and widespread public dissatisfaction with both impersonal medical treatment and the failure of medical technology to deal adequately with chronic illness. The attitude of healthy-mindedness, which James saw as a "rising force" in religious expression at the turn of the century, now, as we near the turn of another century, appears to be rising most dramatically in the area of health care.

There is a striking continuity between the religious and the medical versions of healthy-mindedness. Even in its secularized medical manifestations, the mythos retains a stress on faith and a sense of spirituality that are quasi religious. And it springs from the same buoyant optimism that James describes so well. In health care today, the mythos of healthy-mindedness appears to have three basic and defining aspects. The most important of these is the emphasis on psychological and emotional factors in the cause and treatment of illness. Disease is considered not as a foreign entity that invades the body but a complicated pathological process, whose progress or regress depends upon the patient's psychological constitution and personal response to treatment. The attempt to identify and nurture the life-enhancing aspects of one's self and one's body is here of primary importance. Cure is assumed to come about from the cooperation of external means (radiation, chemotherapy, or changes in diet and exercise) and internal forces—especially, "the will to live." And this "will to live" is conceived not as a psychological abstraction but as a physiological reality, one with genuine therapeutic potential (Cousins 1979, 44).

Also central to healthy-mindedness is a belief in the *vis medicatrix naturae*—the healing power of nature—a Hippocratic concept revised and popularized in recent years by Norman Cousins. The assumption is that the body has the ability to heal itself and that it will do so if certain conditions are maximized, such as maintaining hope and eliminating toxins from one's diet and environment. Along with the belief in the self-healing capacities of the body goes an idealization of nature: anything that is "natural" is good; anything that is a product of technology is suspect. Good food, fresh air, and a life that minimizes stress are thus considered essential to regaining health.

A third characteristic of healthy-mindedness is the emphasis on the active involvement of patients in all aspects of their treatment. The idea that ill persons should be active participants in their therapies can be seen as modernizing and personalizing the older notion that the body has self-healing capacities. Perhaps it is this synthesis of the ancient Hippocratic idea of the healing power of nature with contemporary (and quintessentially American) emphases on the values of self-reliance, individualism, and, perhaps most important, activism, that accounts for the attraction of healthy-mindedness today. Self-assertion in the United States has become itself a bona fide virtue: hence our marked aversion both to passivity in all its forms and to victimization of any kind. Since the word "patient" means one who endures or suffers and is etymologically connected with that dreaded word *passive,* it is not used at all in some discussions of alternative therapies. Bernie Siegel replaces it with *respant,* meaning "responsible participant," a term better denoting the active role of the sick person in the healthy-minded approach to sickness and therapy (1989, 144). The key word for such patient involvement is "responsibility": sick persons are understood to be responsible for incurring their illness, usually by their lifestyle, stress, or feelings of unresolved anger and depression, and they are also responsible for getting well again.

These three characteristics—a positive attitude, the body's capacity to heal itself, and "active" patienthood—are of course interrelated. The assumptions that the body has innate healing capacities and that there is a causal link between mental and physical phenomena liberate sick persons from the role of passive dependence required of a "patient" in the biomedical model, transforming them into active agents whose vigorous participation is essential to energize those mysterious healing forces within.

Healthy-mindedness appears to function as an enabling myth for a great many sick people who write about their illnesses. Perhaps the most salient characteristic of this mythos as it appears in pathography is the extent to which it is empowering. In its emphasis on control and responsibility, healthy-mindedness frees sick persons from dependence on a medical system that is too often depersonalizing, bureaucratic, and uncaring. Regularly, the authors of pathographies informed by this mythos testify to the moment when they achieved freedom and power by taking responsibility for their own treatment. Lucy Shapero, in *Never Say Die,*

comes to this point when her cancer returns eight years after its first appearance: "This time I would make my own decision. Never again would
I listen and automatically obey. . . . I would determine, for myself, what to
do" (86). Ray Berté in his pathography writes that though at first he
"meekly submitted" to a laryngectomy for malignant throat cancer, he later
adopted a "new attitude": "I stopped taking orders and started making
decisions. I stopped thinking of my doctors as gods who would deliver me
from hell and started thinking of them as merely one aspect of my own,
self-designed treatment plan" (11). For Neil Fiore, undergoing treatment
for a tumor near his testicle, the turning point is when *he* determines he
has had enough chemotherapy, requests a tumor board consultation (which
confirms his judgment), and terminates therapy.

Moreover, the healthy-minded approach is empowering in the way it
redefines the doctor-patient relationship. As a consequence of emphasizing
active involvement of the patient in all aspects of therapy, the physician's
role changes to that of a partner, a colleague, and, ideally, a human being
who feels (and shows) genuine respect for the other human being who is
his or her patient. Kenneth Shapiro's advice to his readers on how to deal
with doctors reflects the kind of relationship sought: "Ask questions, know
what to expect. . . . Always keep in mind that you are not only a part of
the team, you are the *most important* part" (124).

The belief that one can actually change the course of illness by maintaining a positive attitude, assuming responsibility for illness, and taking
charge of one's treatment is indeed "strong medicine." But the conviction
that this approach really works is a common motive for writing these pathographies. They are "testimonies," in almost the religious sense. To quote
one cancer patient who attributes her cure to a strict detoxification diet:
"I wrote this account of my experience because I believe that what happened to me is relevant far beyond my individual fate. My own survival
. . . is important as a case history, because it proves that, against all expectations, a highly unconventional, though medically sound, therapy has
succeeded" (Bishop, 12).

The Pathographies

Attitudes and behaviors associated with healthy-mindedness are evident in
many pathographies published in recent years. These books are as varied
as the therapies they describe, but for the sake of clarity, I will organize
them into three groups: (1) the "typical" healthy-minded pathography, in

which the author engages in some form of mind control or alternative therapy as a supplement to orthodox medical treatment—a group I call "psychocentric" pathographies; (2) the "eclectic," a smaller group whose authors sample a great many different kinds of alternative therapy; and (3) the "negative," a still smaller group in which healthy-mindedness can be seen as functioning as a disabling myth. A related though independent group is the pathographies that describe in detail the utilization of a nutritional approach to reverse disease and restore health. The mythic component of these pathographies is problematic because it does not surface in language or imagery; nonetheless, one senses that the thinking behind these pathographies involves an Edenic myth—the return to an uncorrupted state of nature. While this has obvious correlates with the myth of healthy-mindedness, it seems to be the subject for a separate study.[6]

It is important to emphasize that healthy-mindedness is as much praxis as it is interpretation: the myths considered in earlier chapters describe how sick people *understand* their illnesses; healthy-mindedness refers to what they actually *do* about these problems. And precisely because it involves praxis as well as mythos, healthy-mindedness can claim, in addition to the testimony of patients, authorities who explain and justify the approach. In this it is markedly different from the myths discussed in previous chapters. The experts most frequently referred to in pathographical literature are Norman Cousins, Carl and Stephanie Simonton, and Bernie Siegel. It will clarify our analysis of the three kinds of pathographies to begin with these theorists and examine their attitudes toward illness and treatment, discussing pathographies directly associated with them.[7]

Cousins, who joined the UCLA School of Medicine after retiring as editor of the *Saturday Review,* is the author of several books advocating and legitimizing a healthy-minded approach to illness: *Anatomy of an Illness, The Healing Heart,* and *Head First.* The first two books are themselves pathographies, describing a personal experience of illness and the innovative ways in which Cousins manages his treatment for those illnesses; *Head First* is an attempt to provide scientific evidence from the new field of psychoneuroimmunology for his theories about the beneficial effect of a positive attitude in reversing or halting disease.

Cousins is himself the best exemplar of healthy-mindedness in his approach to his own illnesses. Indeed, there is an uncanny resonance between Cousins's way of characterizing himself, as he explains his stance toward illness in his pathographical writings, and William James's description of healthy-mindedness. James, as we have seen, in an echo of the humoral medical psychology of an older era, depicts the healthy-minded as sanguine, cheerful, and hopeful—in direct opposition to the type he calls the sick soul, who by temperament is pessimistic and melancholic. Cousins likewise portrays himself as hopeful and sanguine and contrasts himself to an opposite type of patient. In *Anatomy of an Illness* and *Head First*, Cousins describes an early experience (he was ten years old) when for six months he was hospitalized in a sanitorium for tuberculosis. The patients he observed there seemed to divide themselves into two groups—the "optimists," who believed they would recover from the disease and lead a normal life, and the "realists" who "resigned themselves to a prolonged and even fatal illness" (1979, 155–56).[8] As one might expect, Cousins spontaneously aligns himself with the first group, the optimists: "I couldn't help being impressed with the fact that the boys in my group had a far higher percentage of 'discharged as cured' outcomes than the kids in the other group." He credits the experience at the sanitorium with making him "aware of the power of the mind in overcoming disease" (1979, 156).[9]

A later illness dramatically ratifies this early, instinctive choice and confirms Cousins's perception of himself as one of the healthy-minded. At age thirty-nine, he has what he calls a "crossroads" experience. A cardiogram shows evidence of a "serious coronary occlusion," and he is told he has eighteen months to live. He returns home, where he is greeted by his two small children: "In that instant, I looked down two roads. One road was marked Cardiac Alley, where I would give up everything important to me and try to squeeze out 18 vegetative and melancholy months. The other road was the one I had been traveling. It was one I knew and loved. It might last 18 months or 18 weeks or 18 minutes; but it was my road" (1983, 41). Cousins's response is predictable for one of his temperament: exuberantly he throws his daughters into the air and commences down the path of healthy-mindedness.

If Cousins is himself an exemplar of the healthy-minded approach, he is also probably its most visible proponent. Of his many publications, *Anatomy of an Illness* stands out as the most widely read. The book is in part a pathography, a lively and entertaining account of his successful recovery from ankylosing spondylitis using a logical if fantastic therapy of his own devising—laughter and vitamin C. It begins with the early symptoms of the disease, his hospitalization soon after, and the various tests to which he is subjected in the attempt to diagnose his condition. By the third paragraph of the book, Cousins is already criticizing the hospital: for its inefficiency, its failure to provide proper nutrition, its lack of sanitation, its "promiscuous" use of X-rays and drugs, and its general disregard for the comfort of the patient. Though the hospital earns his scorn, his physician wins his respect as "a man who was able to put himself in the position of the patient" and who "shared my excitement about the possibilities of recovery and liked the idea of a partnership" (30, 39).

Cousins's story of his transition from a hospitalized patient with a serious illness to a sick person who leaves the hospital, researches his condition, and assumes responsibility for his own treatment is worth looking at closely. Musing on the possible causes of his illness, he decides that his immunological defenses were lowered by stress and exposure to pollution during a recent trip to Moscow. His own diagnosis is "adrenal exhaustion," a condition produced by negative emotions and exacerbated by environmental pollutants. He reasons that if negative emotions can so powerfully affect body chemistry for the worse, positive emotions would be likely to produce an equally powerful chemical change for the better. "A plan began to form in my mind for systematic pursuit of the salutary emotions," writes Cousins (35). Immediately he checks himself out of the hospital and moves into a hotel room, substituting vitamin C for anti-inflammatory drugs and replacing painkillers with belly laughs—prompted by watching old "Candid Camera" films and Marx Brothers movies. The results are immediate and dramatic: a much lower sedimentation rate, reduced fever, and a slower pulse. Full recovery, of course, takes some time longer. But after several months, his symptoms abate sufficiently for Cousins to go back to work; and at the time he writes his pathography, he feels his recovery is nearly total (43).

Cousins's book has been enormously popular for people with all kinds of illnesses, often functioning as a handbook to guide them through their experience. It is not hard to understand why this should be so: the author comes across as warm, likeable, and engagingly human; and the book blends optimism, common sense, and a readiness to question and even challenge medical authorities whenever this seems appropriate. But at the same time that one admires the man, commends his approach, and enjoys his story, one may feel the absence of the more profound reflections on illness that might be expected in a book on a subject that is essentially so serious. There is little description of any but the "salutary" emotions: fear, pain, and depression have no place in this pathography. This may seem a weakness, but *Anatomy of an Illness* is virtually a manifesto of healthy-mindedness; and it makes sense that those responses associated with the outlook of the "sick soul" are not represented. For it is the very absence of these darker feelings that signals the success of healthy-mindedness. All such feelings are translated into positive, active measures toward healing.

A useful illustration of Cousins's healthy-minded approach and its influence on patients is *Never Say Die*, a pathography coauthored by Lucy Shapero, a young woman with breast cancer, and Anthony Goodman, a physician, and written ten years after the onset of her symptoms. There are a number of attitudes in this book that reflect a mythology of healthy-mindedness: a doctor-patient relationship based on cooperation and mutual respect, an emphasis on the patient's right to control her therapy, the necessity for self-education in order to exercise that control competently, and the conviction that attitude—the "will to live"—is the most potent of all therapies. The book is especially interesting in the way that it juxtaposes chapters written by the patient with chapters written by the physician. These parallel strands of the experiential and the clinical work well together and are certainly appropriate to the book's central assumption that the best doctor-patient relationship is a cooperative one. Shapero has read Cousins's *Anatomy of an Illness,* a book that has clearly served a formative role in her understanding of her experience: "I had always thought of cancer in terms of conflict: invade, kill, conquer, fight, defend. Cousins spoke of illness in terms of possibility: believe, control, share, hope, protect. I liked that. If I chose life, I preferred to live positively, contributing to and understanding my existence" (132).

Lucy Shapero's story begins when she discovers a lump in her breast. Very soon afterward she undergoes a biopsy and wakes up to discover that a mastectomy has been performed. Later on she learns, with great consternation, that so radical a surgical procedure may not have been necessary. Five years after this, the cancer metastasizes to the cervical spine; it is treated with an ovariectomy and further radiation. Remission this time lasts three years, terminated when a routine bone scan reveals a new spot on the collarbone. Her response now is strong and confident: "This time," she observes, "I would make my own decision. Never again would I listen and automatically obey. I knew where to get information. I knew what books to read. I knew which people to talk to. I would listen, I would study, I would question. And then I would determine, for myself, what to do" (86). This statement seems to epitomize the assertiveness, self-reliance, and insistence on control characteristic of the healthy-minded approach toward illness.

If Cousins's book serves as a model of this approach, inspiring countless patients to educate themselves about their medical condition, question their physicians, become more involved in their treatment, and galvanize the "will to live" into an effective therapeutic force, O. Carl Simonton and Stephanie Matthews-Simonton's *Getting Well Again* suggests practical techniques for encouraging the body to heal itself.[10] A radiation oncologist and a psychotherapist, the Simontons for many years directed a world-famous cancer clinic in Texas, where they advocated the use of relaxation exercises and visualization therapy, in conjunction with traditional medical therapies, as effective treatments for cancer. They maintain that patients who can mobilize positive visual images of white blood cells or chemical agents destroying cancer cells may actually help retard and halt the growth of their cancer. In training the mind to think positively, visualization exercises strengthen the body's natural capacity for healing: the mental joins forces with the physical to form a will to live that is believed to be crucial to the process of recovery. They offer the negative example of a patient who, before therapy, visualizes his cancer as "big black rats" and his treatment as "little yellow pills." Occasionally this patient pictures a rat eating one of these pills and becoming disabled, but such disablement is only temporary (151–52). This imagery of cancer as powerful but treatment as weak and impotent betrays a "negative expectancy" and parallels his deteriorating physical condition. In such a situation, a Simonton patient would be taught to picture the disease cells as chaotic and weak and the therapeutic agents or white blood cells as organized and powerful—as sharks, or piranhas, or knights in white armor. Through relaxation, visualization exercises emphasizing desired outcome, counseling, and if necessary a change of lifestyle, the patient's attitude is modified to one more positive and more hopeful of a cure.

The Simontons preface their description of this technique with theoretical explanation and justification. Most importantly, they indicate that a "central premise" in their approach is the belief "that emotional and mental states play a significant role both in *susceptibility* to disease, including cancer, and in *recovery* from all disease" (10). Stress, recent bereavement, and a personality configuration tending toward feelings of helplessness and depression are important causative factors in the onset of cancer. The therapeutic method derived from these beliefs is based on the assumption "that the cycle of cancer development can be reversed" (95), that hope, belief, and a resolve to recover can positively affect physiological conditions conducive to recovery.

The Simontons' book (or method) is referred to at least as often in pathographies as is *Anatomy of an Illness*. Most commonly, authors mention visualization therapy when they allude to the Simontons' work. A surprising number of patients supplement their orthodox medical treatments with these exercises, creating concrete images of an illness being overcome by its therapeutic antagonists. So one author with cancer writes of her efforts "to imagine my myeloma cells exploding, to visualize the abnormal protein disappearing" (Thompson, 248). Another remarks on her sick husband's attempts in "trying to meditate away his illness, picturing his white blood cells multiplying and the AIDS virus dying" (E. Cox, 72). A third understands visualization exercises as "specifically focusing upon cancer being a weak disease and the cancer cell being a weak, confused, deformed cell" (Ireland, 64).

In pathographies that discuss alternative treatment modalities, visualization therapy is probably the single most common method. Why should this particular practice enjoy such wide popularity? In the first place, it is easy and painless, costs nothing, and entails no risk. Moreover, it follows the logic of wishful thinking—the mythic notion that to want something very, very much is to better one's chances of getting it. But it is compelling for deeper reasons as well, resonating with some of our oldest myths about the human condition. The belief that human life is a perpetual battle between good and evil is just such a myth. So the Simontons see disease as "a physical manifestation of the battle being waged between two parts of the self: the toxic or self-destructive parts and the nurturing or life-sustaining parts" (173). The militant confrontation between evil and good is the stuff of epic both ancient and modern, literary and popular: one thinks of Beowulf fighting Grendel, or, more recently, the battle between Luke Skywalker and Darth Vader. In the Simontons' visualization exercises, the patient intervenes in the epic battle of disease, actively helping the hero (a role played by the white blood cells) defeat the evil predator, cancer. We see how easily the healthy-minded mythos extends to and overlaps with the overtly mythic images and metaphors of warfare discussed in chapter 3.

An interesting extension of visualization therapy is Anne Hargrove's *Getting Better*, a pathography organized around the idea of an "inner guide"—"the person inside you who always tells you the truth"—which she says she has taken from the Simontons' book (21). Most of her pathography is a dialogue between herself and this inner guide, whom she names, fittingly, Carl. Hargrove criticizes her physicians for their emotional remoteness, their evasiveness, and their mechanical optimism. It seems clear that Carl, the inner guide—and Carl Simonton, the author of a book that she clearly finds helpful and meaningful—substitute for the physicians whom she has found deficient. Ironically, the image-therapist himself becomes a therapeutic image.

Most of the patients who engage in Simonton visualization exercises do so as a complement to, not a substitute for, orthodox medical treatment. But many are critical of the medical treatment they receive, faulting their doctors most often for inattention to the nonphysical aspects of an illness. Like Hargrove, Elizabeth Léone Simpson (in a pathography that also cites the influence of the Simontons) criticizes her physicians for failures on the interpersonal level. Hargrove, who assented to a mastectomy and chemotherapy, faults her physicians for their inability to tell the truth and their difficulty in "connecting" with their patients. Simpson, recovering from tubercular meningitis, observes that, though she feels she had "the best medical care available anywhere in the world," her doctors failed her by being emotionally remote: "Learned professional detachment kept these doctors from being emotional resources for me" (107). Given the assumption that mind and body are interrelated (an assumption fundamental to a healthy-minded perspective) and that healing, therefore, necessarily involves mental as well as physical factors, these criticisms address not simply the physician's skill in making a patient feel cared for but also the physician's failure to deal with factors that are believed to influence the course of illness.

A fourth important figure for pathography is Bernie Siegel, a surgeon formerly affiliated with Yale University School of Medicine and the author of two popular books describing an unorthodox approach to cancer treatment. Siegel advocates many of the ideas associated with Cousins and the Simontons, but he goes further. Like them, he emphasizes the ideology of responsibility and control, seeing the patient as necessarily active in all aspects of treatment. For Siegel, not only is illness caused by and symbolic of psychic problems, but it is even a "gift," a catalyst for important and necessary personal change. The onset of disease, then, is the result of an individual's having deviated from the fullest expression of the self, and the avenue to cure lies in returning to the "True Self," which he calls "the DNA of the soul" (1989, 42). The key to actualizing one's life and returning to the true self is love, and this is conceived as a force that the ill person must actively manifest. Siegel calls those capable of this approach "exceptional patients," who "manifest the will to live in its most potent form" (1986, 3). Though he conceives the function of the physician as that of a facilitator—"My role as a surgeon is to buy people time, during which they can heal themselves" (1986, 4)—he is himself a charismatic and powerful force in the lives of those ill people whom he reaches, and his impact implies a more grandiose agenda. His primary and basic interest is healing, in the age-old tradition of those who, through their own charisma, the adoring belief of their followers, or divine agency, restore people to a condition of physical and spiritual well-being. Heal the life, Siegel counsels, and bodily cure will follow.

A pathography illustrating aspects of this approach is Raymond A. Berté's *To Speak Again,* with its one-page introduction by Siegel. Diagnosed as having malignant throat cancer of an unusual kind and treated with a total laryngectomy that leaves him unable to speak, Berté describes his successful struggle to arrest his cancer and adapt to his disability. Responsibility and control are important features in this struggle. Several years later, when told he now has "fourth-stage bone marrow cancer," Berté responds: "I took an aggressive posture, went out and gathered information, and made some decisions" (14). For Berté, healing is for the most part self-healing: he believes that each of us has an inner force that can overcome disabilities of all kinds, and the most important aspect of healing is to learn to harness this force. The body's own resources, which he calls the "internal doctor," are *primary* in healing, though one should not hesitate to turn to physicians when "outside help" is needed. Illness is never accidental; stress, diet, and self-esteem are important contributing factors. And lastly, disease is an opportunity for spiritual growth: Berté feels his cancer experience has actually enhanced his life. This conviction accords with Siegel's idea that disease, properly experienced, is potentially a transformative experience and can, thus, be thought of as a kind of gift.

Berté's position in regard to orthodox medicine seems characteristic of many pathographies that embrace the healthy-minded mythos. He advocates a guarded and careful use of physicians and medical technology, urging his readers "not to abandon traditional medicine, but to be sure to incorporate a holistic approach into their treatment" and warning them not to become "over-reliant on medical technology" (159, 34). His attitude toward physicians is overtly patronizing: he refrains from blaming them for their faults and limitations and, instead, concentrates on helping his readers understand the causes for those flaws. For example, Berté maintains that the reason most physicians do not prescribe vitamins for treatment is because vitamin-therapy is so very effective that it gives patients "power to treat themselves," thereby posing a threat to physicians' need to control their patients. Physicians, Berté implies, are possessed of a neurotic need for power and control over their patients. He qualifies his objections to orthodox medicine with a disclaimer that is genially forgiving and thus lethal: "In spite of my criticisms of the medical profession, I hold physicians in high esteem": after all, doctors are "trained to be 'mechanics,'" and thus it is illogical to expect that they can be anything more. Since Berté has himself assumed the role of healer, his physicians are left the job of mere technicians—a characterization few physicians would accept.

Psychocentric Pathographies: "The Healer Within"

The interactivity of mind and body—an assumption fundamental to healthy-mindedness—makes for a "psychocentric universe" in which psychological factors not only influence recovery but also account for the onset of disease. This conviction gives rise to several ideas found repeatedly in these pathographies: the notion that negative emotions and thoughts are responsible for illness, various ideas about the way attitude can affect the immune and endocrine systems, and the belief that manipulation of attitude can reverse illness.

Pathographers with cancer especially tend to attribute their disease to psychological causes. Alice Hopper Epstein decides that stress and a "cancer-prone personality" were responsible for her illness, Anne Hargrove mentions that she feels her cancer was caused by her trying to be "too good," and David Tate suspects that he may have brought on his cancer by a recurrent suicidal image of himself that occurred during a period of depression some years before. Raymond Berté finds psychological causes not only for the onset of the disease but also for the body part affected, perceiving his throat cancer (and the loss of speech resulting from a laryngectomy) as related to his father's telling him, as a child, that he was too noisy. But it is not only cancer patients who find psychogenic explanations for disease. Elizabeth Léone Simpson sees a stressed and depressed state of mind as a causative factor in her contracting tubercular meningitis; and Mary Kay Blakely, hospitalized for a coma precipitated by flu, locates the cause of her condition in feelings of depression triggered by the recent suicide of her older brother and her own unsatisfactory divorce. Even AIDS, according to George Melton, is a disease reflecting emotional and mental problems.

In pathographies describing all kinds of illnesses, an important part of the author's formulation seems to be the assumption of responsibility for the onset of illness and the recognition of the psychological or behavioral factors that were responsible. This causative link between psyche and soma has mythic origins—most notably in the association of sin and disease so prevalent in earlier Hebraic and Christian cultures. Susan Sontag (among others) believes that the tendency to ascribe psychological causes to diseases like cancer or tuberculosis or AIDS is still very much with us; moreover, she believes this tendency results in the demoralization of an individual already victimized by disease. Unlike Sontag, though, authors of healthy-minded pathographies feel that the association of personality and illness is enabling. Perceiving a link between personal traits and illness affirms a holistic sense of self; and taking responsibility for that link results in an active, involved patient who is determined to reverse the disease process by changing the psychological traits that caused it.

In these pathographies, the author's "confession" of responsibility for illness is most often accompanied by the logical inference that removal of the cause of illness will reverse the course of an illness. Moreover, the site where the psychological is transferred into the somatic, and vice versa, is often thought to be the immune or the endocrine system. Thus if negative emotions have compromised the body's immune system, then positive emotions will restore the body's immunity and result in healing. We remember that Norman Cousins, determining that stress and exposure to pollution caused his illness by weakening his immunological defenses, reasons that laughter and control are likely to strengthen his immunological system and thus restore him to health.

Alice Hopper Epstein, in her pathography about cancer, also emphasizes the link between psychological cause and psychological cure. Diagnosed as having inoperable cancer of the kidney that has metastasized to her lungs, and given three months to live, she is told that the only possible form of treatment is an experimental interferon program. At this point, she and her husband begin to research alternative forms of cancer therapy. In particular, she mentions the books of Siegel, the Simontons, and Cousins as influential in teaching her about the psychological dimensions of her illness. Epstein attributes the onset of cancer to two factors: the stress of studying for her Ph.D. exams and a lifelong tendency toward helplessness and self-negation—traits that she feels constitute a "cancer-prone personality." She then offers the "hopeful corollary" that a disease brought on by stress and a cancer-prone personality can be reversed by "the psychological methods that worked for me" (3–5). At first she tries the Simontons' visualization therapy, then various meditation techniques, both Eastern and Western. Eventually she arrives at psychosynthesis, a therapy that uses extensive visualization to create and name "subpersonalities" and then imagine their behavioral responses. Much of her pathography consists of the words and actions of these subselves as they act out the drama of unconscious impulses and compulsions. By understanding in this way the source of the negative feelings that led to her contracting cancer, she is able to work through those feelings—"reversing . . . the cancer-prone personality as it had developed in me" (198).

A psychogenic understanding of illness not only affects patients' explanations of its cause and cure but can also influence whether or not they will accept certain treatments recommended by their doctors. We recall Kenneth Shapiro's belief in "the human immunological system" as "the answer to every disease in the world" (53). This belief dictates his choice of treatment: he reasons that "we should build up the immunologic system and support and encourage it rather than tear it down," and thus he rejects both chemotherapy and radiation in favor of immunotherapy (62). Moreover, Shapiro is convinced that "the patient *must* believe in his or her treatment and have full confidence in it in order for it to work" (99). Since he has no confidence in chemotherapy or radiation, he feels justified in refusing them. A second example is Max Lerner, who in *Wrestling with the Angel* describes a similar decision about treatment. When Lerner's doctors disagree whether to add radiation therapy to the chemotherapy he has already received for advanced large cell lymphoma—a therapy that he has supplemented with visualization exercises—Lerner casts the deciding vote against it, remarking that "while I had an imagery for the battle of the cells, I had none for radiation" (71).

George Melton's *Beyond AIDS* exemplifies all the features we have been tracing in psychogenic pathographies. The parallel between cause and cure of disease is particularly strong here. Certain beliefs, Melton explains, produce corresponding emotions, and these in turn activate the endocrine system to produce health or illness. He reasons that if the emotional problems that caused the disease are corrected, the disease will simply disappear. "AIDS," he remarks, was "a message from my body. . . . the greatest teacher about life I had ever encountered" (54). Melton believes that love is a therapeutic agent crucial to his recovery. His justification for this conviction beautifully illustrates the interaction between mind and body so central to healthy-mindedness. He begins with the idea of the centrality of the endocrine system in determining health or illness, which he further develops in his belief that "the glands of the endocrine system correspond to the seven chakras in the body" (101). More specifically, the thymus gland, which nurtures the T-cells destroyed by AIDS, is the physical correlate to the heart chakra and is activated by love (132). Melton's notion of love as a potent therapeutic agent is the determining principle in his decision to discontinue treatment. Deciding that the AIDS virus "was not really the enemy" but that "the walls and defenses I had built around myself that kept love out were the only real enemies I had," Melton stops taking his medication (68). It is a decision that he feels is successful: by the end of the book, he sees himself as an "AIDS survivor."

The key to recovery from illness, according to these pathographies, is the act of energizing the will to live. As one author observes, "Medicine, by itself, just is not enough. The will to live must be the overriding, powerful source of your fight" (Shapiro, 124). For the most part, the authors of these pathographies do use orthodox medicine and view the various ways of energizing the will to live as a supplement (though a necessary supplement) to mainstream medical therapy. But many, as we have noted, are critical of the medical care they have received, often faulting their physicians for being impersonal, detached, and uncaring. For this reason, these authors appear to be extremely wary of medical care they might need in the future: their physicians seem potential threats as much as potential helpers. The belief in the "inner healer," an inborn healing potential that the patient must learn to activate in order to recover, is a mythic solution to this problem of the needed though distrusted doctor. It is also central to the healthy-minded pathographies in the next section, a group that differs from those just discussed primarily in the number and quantity of alternative therapies with which the author experiments.

The Eclectic Pathographies: "Shopping for a Cure"

In most of the pathographies described so far, the authors seem cautious, even thoughtful, in their choice of alternative therapies. Others, in contrast, seem to be characterized by an unrestrained, exuberant, sometimes even playful tendency to sample a wide variety of treatment modalities in the search for a cure. Jill Ireland's *Life Wish* provides a useful introduction to this second group of healthy-minded pathographies. Early in the narrative, Ireland discovers she has breast cancer, which is treated with a mastectomy and chemotherapy. But she feels that the medical therapies by themselves are not sufficient. She listens to tapes describing the Simontons' technique of meditation and visualization exercises and even sees Simonton himself for individual counseling sessions. Meditation, she observes, "gave me a task, something I could do alone to get myself well. . . . The energy was there waiting to be tapped. It knew what to fight" (77). However, the question of just how to tap this potential for healing seems in her case—as in that of others—to lead to an escalating search for better or different catalysts. Ireland turns to a holistic doctor, who has her drink, eight times a day, an electrically charged fluid and gives her biweekly "table treatments," in which she lies on a table fitted up with "electromagnetic wave vibrations to rebalance my body's cells" (77). From this she moves on to try acupuncture, astrology, and quartz crystals. There is little indication that she understands the systems of Chinese and American Indian medicine from which acupuncture and the use of quartz crystals derive, and astrology, she admits, is something she does as a diversion.[11] Her decision to try these therapies appears to be motivated not so much by belief in the treatment as by the sense that it cannot hurt and by a conviction that she should be doing something about getting well.

One question that might be raised at this point is whether the tendency to sample various therapies is generated by a sense of frustration and even despair with an orthodox medical approach, whether it represents "good problem solving" when dealing with a disease for which biomedicine has only limited therapeutic resources, or whether it is simply a dimension of our national consumerism, with its assumption that more is always better. The growing incidence of such experimentation with alternative therapies may point to certain important changes in our attitude as a culture toward both sickness and orthodox medicine.

First, as I suggested at the beginning of this chapter, health care has indeed become a commodity, at least for those who are in a position to afford it. We are a nation of shoppers, and ill people today often feel it appropriate to "shop around" for a therapy they feel suits them best. As one author remarks about her choice of treatment, "I had done my market research, inspected the goods and asserted my right to a free choice. All I had to do now was to decide what to buy" (Bishop, 101).[12] Second, the tendency toward large-scale experimentation with alternative treatments suggests that many people have decided that orthodox medicine is inadequate.[13] If sickness affects the whole person, as advocates of healthy-mindedness assume, and if orthodox medicine defines itself as strictly concerned with disease as a biochemical phenomenon, then the pursuit of alternative medical therapies for these people is a logical consequence. In short, the rise of alternative medicine may reflect a cultural consumerism where medicine has become a commodity and also a cultural dissatisfaction with biomedicine both in theory and in practice.

Given this dissatisfaction, it is surprising that *none* of these authors who recount their search for a cure describes doctors, hospitals, or medical procedures with the anger and resentment that characterize some pathographies. Ireland, for example, appears to have good relationships with all her doctors, and her hospital experience seems free from the depersonalizing treatment about which so many authors complain. Not only is she a compliant patient, but even while she is dabbling in various forms of alternative therapies, her attitude toward her own physicians (and toward orthodox medicine) remains extremely positive. Why, then, does she turn to alternative medicine? It appears that she does so as a necessary complement to orthodox medicine, having recognized and accepted its limitations. Medical science had done its part, she observes, and now she must do hers: "It was time for me to discover why I had become sick" (73). Ireland, like the authors whose books are described below, simply wants to cover all the bases. As she observes, "I wanted the best of all worlds: the AMA, my homeopathic healer, and my holistic therapists" (137).

Often in these pathographies, the search for a cure seems to become the content and purpose of one's life. In *Health, Hope, and Healing,* the author's initial attempt to find a cure for his illness turns into a search for self-fulfillment. David Tate, diagnosed as having stage II Hodgkin's disease (at a time when this disease had a poor prognosis), complements radiation treatments and chemotherapy with various alternative therapies. Believing that the will to live is the key to recovery but feeling that he must do more than just assert this desire, Tate determines that he needs to "reclaim his dreams." He had always wanted to be a psychotherapist, and now he goes back to school and earns his accreditation; he had always wished to be a stand-up comic, and by the end of the narrative, he has become this too.

Through the course of the pathography, Tate describes his experiences with a variety of alternative medical practices: meditation, Silva Mind Control (verbal affirmations and visual imagery), the remedies of Edgar Cayce (castor oil packs, osteopathic manipulations, and a positive attitude), acupuncture, psychic healing, out of body experiences, lucid dreaming (the ability to remain lucid throughout a dream and direct its outcome), transpersonal psychology, and psychosynthesis (a Jungian form of image-therapy). This part of the narrative concludes with his becoming a comedian—the apex of his transformation and the realization of his deepest dreams. Well before the book ends, it becomes clear that what Tate is pursuing is no longer a cure for Hodgkin's disease but self-realization. The illness, he feels, has served as the catalyst for major transformations in every aspect of his life.

The habit of sampling alternative therapies, often combining them with orthodox medical treatment, is not only characteristic of cancer patients. An example is *Thanksgiving,* by Elizabeth Cox, a pathography describing the illness and death of her husband, Keith, from AIDS. While receiving orthodox medical treatment, Keith sees a psychiatrist "who specializes in AIDS victims" and a nutritionist, listens to Simonton imagery tapes, and consults by mail a Tibetan doctor in India. The Tibetan treatment is at first carried on long distance: Keith sends a urine sample and in return receives some pills. Later on, however, the Tibetan doctor actually appears on the scene. Unfortunately, the author tells us little about this doctor or his therapies, though treatment with him is continued throughout Keith's illness. It is of interest that the Coxes consult the Tibetan doctor as to the advisability of mixing Eastern and Western remedies, but they never tell their Western physician of his Eastern counterpart. Pathographies suggest that this tendency not to tell orthodox doctors about alternative treatments is widespread.

For Cox, and many others, alternative medical therapies function as a supplement to orthodox medicine. But in George Melton's pathography about AIDS, discussed earlier for its emphasis on psychological aspects of illness, little reference at all is made to doctors or to any aspect of traditional medical care (though we are told, incidentally, of regular visits to a physician). This pathography is not characterized by noncompliance or by any sort of negativity or criticism of doctors and hospitals; instead, medicine is simply relegated to a peripheral status.

The book begins when both the author and his lover, Wil, are diagnosed as having ARC. Understanding that the medical establishment can offer no real help, both men feel free to turn to their own resources in treating their condition. They begin by acquiring Isoprinosine from a friend. But when subsequent medical tests indicate the onset of Kaposi's sarcoma for Wil and a depressed T-cell count for Melton, they determine to take more drastic measures. At first they travel to Mexico and smuggle the illegal drug Ribavirin back into the country, but their approach changes when they read the Simontons' *Getting Well Again* and the writings of trance channel Edgar Cayce. "Awakened" to the connection between mind and body, falsely separated "in current medical thought" (38), they give up smoking and alcohol and commence upon a program of prayer, nutrition, and weekly massages. Greatly impressed by the ideas of a disembodied presence named Seth, which have been transmitted through the writer-medium Jane Roberts, Melton forms a study group to explore the Seth material and "appl[y] what we were learning to our ARC diagnosis" (49). This group experiments with healing crystals, channeling, automatic writing, UFOs and extraterrestrials, and the manipulation of dreams—"lucid dreaming." By this point, Melton has stopped taking any medication, and he and Wil both decide they do not want to know the results of the T-cell tests that they submit to regularly. Both men feel not only that their illness is cured as a result of these varied therapies but that their lives have been enhanced in the process. AIDS, writes Melton, enabled him to "realign" his beliefs and life-style to a more spiritually centered sense of life (54).

Laura Chester's pathography about lupus is also impressive for the number and variety of therapies that the author tries in her search for a cure. But whereas Melton seems almost oblivious to orthodox medicine, Chester sometimes combines and sometimes oscillates between orthodox and alternative medical therapies. Chester is married, thirty-one years old, and the mother of two young children when her symptoms first begin. She consults a rheumatologist, who treats her symptoms with aspirin and then prednisone as her condition worsens. Though her relationship with the rheumatologist appears to be a good one, she decides to complement orthodox therapy with other forms of treatment. She turns to anthroposophical medicine, a homeopathic system derived from the theories of Rudolf Steiner. Her treatment consists of curative eurythmy (a movement therapy) and injections of Iscador, a mistletoe derivative. When her condition continues to worsen, she tries Gerson therapy (a detoxification diet) and weekly acupuncture treatments. When these do not help, she returns to prednisone and plaquenil, whereupon her condition does improve. But she has difficulty with the side effects of these drugs.

Midway through her narrative, deciding that she wants something more than management of her disease, she declares: "I felt like it was time to start seeking a cure" (73). The search described in the rest of the book differs only in degree, not in kind, from the combination of orthodox and alternative medical therapies described in the first part. From homeopathic and allopathic medicine she determines "to take what each could offer" (74). And this is precisely what she does. She consults a healer, attends lectures given by the American Lupus Society, seeks out a massage therapist trained in Ortho-Bionomy who gives her the Bach Flower-Remedies, attends kundalini yoga sessions at a nearby ashram, and sees a chiropractor. During all this, she visits her doctor regularly, her lupus in remission.

Moving to another part of the country, she continues her efforts to achieve a cure, finding another anthroposophical doctor who puts her on a special diet, prescribes birch-leaf tea, rosemary baths, digestives, and certain minerals to be taken in conjunction with the waxing and waning of the moon. In addition, he has her take injections in the stomach of Formica, a derivative of red ants, because "red ants are incredibly quick at bringing dead matter back into the life cycle" (133). She also sees a therapist skilled in psychosynthesis. Again she combines these approaches with orthodox treatment, finding herself a rheumatologist whom she sees regularly. At the end of her pathography, Chester knows that she is not "cured" of lupus, but she feels that her efforts have succeeded in keeping it in remission. Though she allows that orthodox medicine, in the form of prednisone, did once come to her rescue, she attributes her success in maintaining that remission primarily to the combined effects of anthroposophical medicine and psychosynthesis therapy. In the years to come, she imagines herself "healthy, yet always on the alert, watching for symptoms, continuing my homeopathic remedies, growing stronger, less afraid, more relaxed" (170).

I have discussed these "eclectic" pathographies in detail so that the reader will have some sense of the richness and variety of the therapies they describe. It is worth pointing out that there is no one type of patient or disease characteristic of this group: they include a movie star with breast cancer, a young attorney with Hodgkin's disease, two men with AIDS, and a young mother with lupus. In reading these pathographies, one is struck partly by the bizarreness of the combinations of treatments; also by the ease with which health care is treated as a commodity and pursued as such. Orthodox medicine is but one of several "brands" available.

Negative Pathographies: "Some Poems Don't Rhyme"

We tend to be attracted to healthy-mindedness precisely because it is life-affirming, optimistic, and hopeful in the face of illnesses that are painful, debilitating, and often fatal. A healthy-minded approach is to an illness such as cancer, or lupus, or AIDS as David is to Goliath, and its tools are often analogous to that biblical slingshot and pebble. We cheer the efforts of our "Davids" in fighting these illnesses, and when the pebble does hit the mark, we all applaud.

But like other myths about illness, healthy-mindedness has its negative side, too. This mythos has by now become so entrenched that it already has its detractors in pathographical literature. So Paul Monette, writing about AIDS, takes offense at "the growing 'empowerment' movement," with its assumptions about the sick person's responsibility for incurring illness and capacity to bring about a cure through right attitude. He dismisses the approach as "the whole guilt-and-redemption trip" (227). As we have seen, Monette chooses the battle theme, not healthy-mindedness, as the organizing myth of his pathography. For Monette, AIDS is more than a disease; it represents a biological version of his culture's persecution of homosexuality. Thus, the proper response for the person afflicted with AIDS is to fight the disease, just as the proper response for the AIDS community is to fight homophobia. AIDS is here understood as solely a physical disorder, and its cure is expected to come about through medical science: a promising drug has "the status of a Holy Grail in the AIDS underground" (196), and some final cure or "magic bullet" is expected at any moment.

Monette, then, rejects the healthy-minded mythos because its ideology of responsibility and control is dystonic with his acceptance of his homosexuality. Barbara Webster, who suffers from multiple sclerosis, also finds healthy-mindedness unhelpful. She shares Monette's distaste for the idea that "failure to overcome the disease flows in large part from defects in character and will" (27) and feels that the tendency of popular books about illness (especially pathographies) to focus on overcoming or conquering disease is counterproductive for patients with a chronic, incurable disease such as hers. The emphasis such writings place on hope, optimism, and positive thinking can make it difficult for these patients to accept the changes and limitations imposed by their illness: in such popular literature, she observes, hope "is used as a way around reality" and seems "to obviate the need for acceptance, foreclose the need to deal with reality, and support denial" (29). A "full acceptance of present reality and potential consequences," she argues, is preferable to the optimistic outlook advocated by the healthy-minded approach (28).

Monette and Webster are critical of healthy-mindedness, but they are distanced from it: the mythos is not one that shapes their own personal experiences of illness. However, there are pathographies that demonstrate the disabling potential of this optimistic, hopeful, life-affirming mythos. And there are indeed problems with healthy-mindedness, some of them rather obvious. First, it is often impractical: the kind of competence expected of patients, if they are to make important decisions about their treatment, depends on the availability of up-to-date educational materials, the intelligence to understand them, and the willingness to discard approaches that are medically unsound. Second, the training of physicians today does not encourage a fully cooperative relationship with patients, and thus it may be difficult to find a doctor who is both medically competent and sympathetic to this kind of therapeutic alliance. Third, the mythos is psychologically naive: an individual's basic attitude, which is crucial here, is not so easily controlled or changed. Fourth, it is a mythos that is particularly dangerous for those patients whose illness does not reverse itself, whose efforts to affirm life and believe in themselves only culminate in death.

The mythos of healthy-mindedness can be as deceptive as it is attractive. In Virginia Hine's *Last Letter to the Pebble People,* discussed in the preceding chapter as an example of "transcendent death," healthy-mindedness seems to produce a disabling effect. Aldie Hine is fifty-four years old when he discovers he has cancer. Midway through life he had turned, somewhat unsuccessfully, from a flourishing though personally unfulfilling career in business to a career as a marine biologist. Throughout the narrative there are statements indicating that the family sees Aldie as having failed in this new career to live up to his potential.

Aldie's illness begins with certain symptoms that he intuitively and correctly diagnoses as lung cancer. After a visit to his doctor, he consents to a five-week period of radiation treatment, which the family supplements with the combined "energy forces" generated by a large number of people meditating simultaneously. The "statement of hope" that the family sends out to potential meditators is virtually a manifesto of the healthy-minded approach: "WE BELIEVE that energy forces for healing, beyond present medical knowledge, exist and can be tapped if many people join their thoughts and love together for this purpose. We think that the power of focused love can 'irradiate' the body in cooperation with the cobalt beam" (27–28). Practically, this endeavor consists of the formation of a network of some two hundred individuals who agree to meditate at the same time each day, the theme being Aldie's recovery. Those who are in the area gather together near a fountain at the Hines' home, where they signal their membership in this therapeutic community by throwing a pebble into the pool; those who live far away are requested to send a pebble that others then deposit in the pool—hence the "Pebble People" of the book's title.

The combined physical and meditative therapies prove successful, resulting in a remission that is believed to be a miraculous cure. It is during this remission that the Hines visit the Simonton cancer clinic in Fort Worth with the intent of strengthening Aldie's ability to remain healthy through focused mental imagery. One of the assumptions of the Simontons' approach to illness, as the author understands it, is that in certain individuals "there is a pattern of responses, a mental and emotional orientation or a life-style, which creates the conditions for cancer as a response to certain life situations" (36). The Hines enthusiastically embrace the ideology of control and responsibility and link it retrospectively to their initial success in combining meditation and radiation: "The power of the Pebble People network," writes the author, "enabled [Aldie] to become strong enough to begin to accept responsibility for his own disease" (34).

But as the author herself observes, "The concept of responsibility in self-healing can be a double-edged sword" (54). Several months later, Aldie discovers a small node in his groin and another near the right collarbone. He determines that this new development should be treated by utilizing mind control as the sole therapeutic medium.[14] Thus he does not pursue medical treatment but, instead, intensifies his efforts "to pour energy into his body's fight against the cancer" (40). But the nodes continue to grow.

Aldie returns to Fort Worth for two intensive days of counseling with the Simontons, where he experiences an intuitive realization that he is going to die. With this realization, the Hines reach toward a stance that will permit them to accept the inevitability of his dying. As they struggle to accept the death that both know to be imminent, they still cast about "for some radical change in . . . lifestyle that would reverse the course of the disease" (52). Thus they embark on a ten-day stay at Swami Rama's Himalayen Institute. However, hatha yoga, meditation, and a vegetarian diet fail to alleviate Aldie's condition, and the Hines again return to the Simonton clinic, where Aldie accepts radiation treatments to reduce his pain.

There are difficulties in the transition from the controlling and self-reliant ideology of responsibility, which husband and wife had found so helpful during the phase of illness, to the gentler and quieter attitude of acceptance. The difficulty seems to arise from the inappropriateness of the healthy-minded mythos, with its aggressive, assertive, controlling sensibility, to the task of dying, which may be made easier by adopting what earlier generations referred to as "the passive virtues"—acceptance, surrender, the ability to let go. Whereas earlier Aldie had been expected to participate actively in his own therapy—focusing the power of the "will to live" toward healing—what is required of him now is the ability to confront and accept his own death.

Still, the Hines cling to the healthy-minded mythos. Having failed to control his illness, they turn their energies toward controlling his dying. Husband and wife at this point issue a manifesto that begins: "We commit ourselves to an active participation in our own death process. We choose to die at home, not in a hospital. We intend to have full choice over the place and method of death" (43). This document is remarkable in the way the ideology of responsibility and control has been displaced in its entirety from illness onto dying.

Healthy-mindedness is further adapted to the task of dying in the notion of "victorious death." For some people, the author observes, "a victorious death" occurs gratuitously, as the natural consequence of "deeper levels of their life patterns." But for Aldie, "a victorious death seems to require an intense period of very intentional training" (12). One cannot help wondering if Aldie's failure to reverse his illness is not responsible, at least in part, for the demands made upon him as he approaches death. Indeed, there are references throughout the book to a passivity in Aldie's character that his wife sees as contributing both to his contracting cancer and to his failure to reverse the illness: "There was about him such a sense of unfulfilled potential. . . . if Aldie would only grasp the power of his potential and fling himself into its fulfillment, he would be saved" (66). To see dying as the supreme and telic opportunity for self-realization does indeed rescue the earlier emphasis on responsibility and right attitude, but at a heavy human cost. Death here becomes not simply the end of a life but its very purpose, and the quality of life is judged by the heroism that is seen to accrue to the act of dying itself—a heroism bordering on sanctity.

A very real problem with the mythos of healthy-mindedness, as this narrative demonstrates, is that it can engender guilt on the part of the ill person and blame on the part of loved ones. For a corollary of the notion that attitude affects illness is the belief that when an individual does not succeed in reversing the course of illness it is because he or she did not try hard enough—or did not really want to. The author's insistence that her husband can recover, if only he tries hard enough, is later transformed into an acceptance of his dying that makes death itself an arena for self-realization: so she observes that it was "[Aldie's] unrealized potential that made death the only viable alternative to a future half-life half lived" (68).

Gilda Radner's pathography, though it does not actually end with her death, also demonstrates the disabling potential of the mythos of healthy-mindedness. Known to the American public from her outrageously comic impersonations on "Saturday Night Live," Radner also gained a wide audience by publishing the story of her cancer experience, *It's Always Something*. Throughout the narrative, Radner, the author, is consistent with Radner, the comedienne, in affirming the archetypically comic principles of hope, love, and life over their tragic counterparts—despair, loneliness, and death. Characteristically, her pathography begins not with the initial symptoms of her disease but with a long and happy reminiscence about the early days of her relationship with her husband. "Like in the romantic fairy tales I always loved, Gene Wilder and I were married by the mayor of a small village in the south of France, September 18, 1984" (15). This is the first sentence of her pathography—as fine an expression of the archetypically comic as one is likely to find: the colloquial and ungrammatical "like" suggesting the triumph of irreverence and spontaneity over a sober and rule-bound syntax, the setting romantic and yet down to earth, the image of a storybook wedding affirming the theme of love and romance successfully realized in marriage. But the happy ending of comedy is only the beginning of this pathography.

The theme of illness works its way into the narrative gradually, and relatively late, beginning with symptoms of fatigue and a vague malaise. Radner is prompt in seeking medical advice, but internist, gastroenterologist, and gynecologist all fail to arrive at a correct diagnosis for her problems. And so does she, convinced that the diagnoses they give of Epstein-Barr virus and mittelschmerz are "fitting diseases for the Queen of Neurosis" (52). Frustrated, she visits an acupuncturist and then a holistic doctor, who advocates coffee enemas and protein supplements; perhaps more important, the holistic therapist calls her daily to find out how she is feeling. Radner concludes that acupuncturist and holistic therapist, unlike her orthodox doctors, are "taking me seriously" and "paying attention to me" (66) and that this justifies her turning to them for treatment. At one point, suffering from severe stomach pains, she visits three different kinds of therapist within a five-day period: the acupuncturist sticks needles in her stomach and gives her an abdominal massage, the holistic doctor suggests a colonic to clean out the bowel, the internist gives her a gamma globulin shot and a prescription for laxatives. Radner here admits to a superfluity of therapists and treatments, and raises the question as to whether or not she should "tell the doctors about each other." Apparently, she does not. Instead, she chooses between them, deciding on the holistic doctor because he "was paying the most attention to me" (67).[15]

Eventually her symptoms reach a point at which hospitalization becomes necessary. When tests finally reveal that she has ovarian cancer, Radner consents to an immediate hysterectomy and subsequent chemotherapy. Again she turns to alternative treatment modalities, but this time as complements to, rather than substitutes for, orthodox medical treatment. At the advice of her oncologist, she sees a therapist specializing in relaxation and visualization exercises. Finding this helpful, she goes on to join a cancer support group, which instructs participants in guided imagery and relaxation and teaches them how to "take control of their recovery." She begins wearing healing crystals "as reminders of the body's and the spirit's desire and capacity to be well" (174). She makes up a chant— "I am well, I am wonderful, I am cancer-free"—which she uses as much to drive out negative thoughts as to affirm the positive: "I'd have these words to think so that the cancer thoughts couldn't get in." She finds herself smiling as she repeats this chant, remarking: "I knew that smiling a lot helps fight disease" (178). Despite the nausea, hair loss, and fatigue she experiences as side effects of the chemotherapy, her spirits are high.

At this point her narrative changes direction. She agrees to a second-look surgery, though she worries "that if they did find more cancer. . . . it would destroy my faith in my own sensibility and my sense about my body" (181). Unfortunately, the biopsy reveals "two microscopic cancer cells," and her physicians want her to begin another round of chemotherapy. She is crushed by this result, "totally shattered" and "terribly depressed," and the healthy-minded approach begins to backfire: "I couldn't deal with the premise that after you have done everything right, done everything you could possibly do—positive thinking, crystals, visualization, psychotherapy, gotten your head into a wonderful place, everything—suddenly it turns out that perfect behavior might not have worked" (191, 194). To make matters worse, Radner has even "gone public" with her assertion of the value of hopefulness and a positive attitude: she has been on the cover of *Life* magazine as "a symbol of conquering cancer . . . a symbol of getting well . . . a model cancer patient completely active in [her] own therapy." And now, she concludes, "I felt like a living example that it didn't work" (228, 231).

Radner deals with this new stage of her illness at first by combining chemotherapy and macrobiotics. The therapists for each kind of treatment are starkly contrasted: they emerge in the narrative as life and death, hope and despair; one wears the mask of comedy, the other that of tragedy. The macrobiotic counselor restores her optimism and her good spirits when he assures her that she has a chance to recover: she quips, "That was the best news I'd heard in forever" (237–38). But the oncologist withholds the hope she so desperately craves: "All I could see in the Connecticut oncologist's face was that he didn't believe I would recover. He seemed to have no hope for me, and I had no faith in him" (238). Here the medical "gaze," instead of offering comfort and compassion, only exacerbates her suffering. "That doctor," she observes, "is death to me. He looks at me and he sees me dying" (243). Not unpredictably, she walks out on the oncologist. But despite a frantic and slavish adherence to a macrobiotic life style (she even has a live-in macrobiotic cook), complemented by sessions on psychic healing and a series of interviews with the holistic therapist Lawrence LeShan, her condition does not improve. Once again she changes therapies, terminating the macrobiotic diet and returning to an orthodox cancer specialist to begin another course of chemotherapy—a treatment that she is told has an eighty-five-percent chance of success. Radner interprets this possibility as a cure: "He was talking about restoring my future, not just prolonging my life. . . . he believes that I will get completely well" (256, 266). She is elated with so generous an offer of hope and soon goes off the macrobiotic diet. At the end of her narrative she is on maintenance chemotherapy, still hopeful of recovery.

Radner concludes her pathography by wryly acknowledging that she wrote the book "with the ending in place before there even *was* an ending" (268). Of course this was to be a happy ending, a perfect ending, one that would resonate with the book's happy beginning: "I wanted to be able to write on the book jacket: 'Her triumph over cancer' or 'She wins the cancer war'" (268). These are, of course, the very titles one finds on the book jackets of a good many healthy-minded pathographies. But as Radner reflects, "Some poems don't rhyme, and some stories don't have a clear beginning, middle and end" (268). She actually concludes with a joke about a maimed dog—an appropriate ending for a book about a disease introduced as "probably the most unfunny thing in the world" (12). Several months after completing her pathography, she dies.

Though Radner's pathography differs from Hine's in that it is written by the ill person herself rather than by the surviving spouse, both books show how healthy-mindedness can prove problematic or even disabling when the course of an illness does not abate or reverse itself. We are given a vivid and detailed picture in Radner's narrative of what we can only infer in the Hine pathography: the crippling disappointment that ensues when a sick person does everything possible to create and maintain a positive attitude and yet her condition worsens. But the two pathographies differ in their attitudes towards death. Whereas the Hines transfer the need for responsibility and control to the work of dying, Radner throughout the narrative resists the thought that she might die from her cancer. "Right from the beginning," she remarks, "I believed that I would get well. I always saw myself surviving" (228). Elsewhere she admits: "I could never deal with death—the fact that people do die of cancer. I blocked it out of my mind. I saw cancer as a battle, as a hell, as tortures, whatever, but you didn't die from it" (217).

If the problems in the Hine narrative stem from a basic incompatibility between healthy-mindedness and the work of dying, the problems in Radner's pathography derive from an insistence on maintaining hope that, paradoxically, leads to an ever escalating desperation. Hope is indeed a powerful therapeutic agent, as wise physicians of all kinds have long recognized. But a healthy-minded approach tends to fetishize this therapeutic virtue, sometimes with disastrous consequences. Gilda Radner is virtually a "hope addict," willing to accept almost any therapy if it offers her some promise of recovery. Her decision to terminate chemotherapy in favor of a macrobiotic treatment turns on this issue: she perceives the macrobiotic counselor she consults as offering her hope—"and all I had to do was cook miso soup a certain way on my gas stove and eat rice cream five or six times a day"—in contrast to the oncologist, who "seemed to have no hope for me" (238). But unrealistic expectations as to cure are not solely the province of alternative medicine. For, in the same way, Radner abandons the macrobiotic treatment for another, different regimen of chemotherapy (and another oncologist) because she feels it offers her the same sense of promise: "He was so positive, he was offering me hope. . . . He believes that I will get completely well" (255, 266). Her craving for hope does keep her in treatment, of one kind or another, but it also prevents her from coming to terms with the very real possibility of death. She cannot envisage that her story may have a tragic outcome.

From beginning to end, Radner is a comedienne, and the humor in this book acts as a poignant and heroic counterpoint to the theme of illness and its gradual triumph. But the insistent tone of hopefulness becomes ever more shrill as the book and the illness near a conclusion: indeed, Radner's experience borders on a despair paradoxically generated by her investment in cultivating a positive attitude. The result of this vicious cycle is a desperate need for hope of unrealistic proportions. As she herself writes, "I was caught in a never-never land of hope and faith in something—maybe a miracle" (260–61).

The Hine pathography shows us how healthy-mindedness can turn from an enabling to a disabling myth within the dynamics of a marital relationship, whereas Radner's pathography demonstrates problems with this mythos that can derive from individual temperament. As we have seen, Radner's healthy-mindedness leads to an obsessive, near-pathological reliance on hope—an obsession fueled by her difficulty in accepting the fact that people do die of cancer and unwittingly reinforced by doctors who evade the truth about the likelihood that the therapies they advocate will reverse her condition. Though hope is certainly important, there are dangers if either patient or physician uses it as an opiate. Radner's pathography shows us that there is no guarantee that a positive attitude, accepting responsibility, and an active involvement in treatment will produce the happy ending typical of comedy. Indeed, it suggests that a patient's anguish may actually be increased by this assumption.

But it would be misleading to conclude on this negative note. Though these last four "negative" pathographies demonstrate that a healthy-minded approach to illness is not helpful for everyone, this mythos does seem to have genuine therapeutic and personal value for most of the people who write about it; indeed, many of these pathographies are intended as testimonies to the helpfulness of such attitudes and practices. A healthy-minded approach, with its active, involved, even feisty patient, does appear to improve the quality of life during illness. And the quality of life during treatment is important not just on humanitarian grounds but for practical reasons as well: a patient who is in great physical pain or discomfort as a result of treatment and who is depersonalized by the manner and setting in which such treatment occurs may well have a diminished chance for survival.

Healthy-mindedness is significant not just for what it offers to those who ascribe to it but also for what it can tell us about the problems of orthodox medicine today. It is possible that the remarkable popularity of this mythos, along with its practical realization in alternative medical therapies, may signal the beginnings of a Kuhnian "paradigm shift" in medicine. Many feel that the emphasis in orthodox medicine on the technological and the biochemical has by now become so exaggerated as nearly to obliterate the actuality of the experiencing patient. So we are willing to spend millions on finding a scientific cure for cancer or AIDS, but we allocate only paltry sums to relieve the misery of the many people who actually die from these diseases. Similarly, our system of medical education is awesome in its scientific training but scandalous in the minimal attention given to the humanistic dimensions of medical practice.

Healthy-mindedness redresses this imbalance in contemporary orthodox medicine. In its assumption that attitude is an important therapeutic agent, its conviction that the ill person must be actively involved in all aspects of treatment, and its redefinition of the role of the physician as partner, healthy-mindedness seriously challenges our medical orthodoxy. If the challenge goes ignored, then biomedicine is likely to become only one of many possible modalities of health care in an increasingly pluralistic society—a modality whose narrow focus on the biochemical aspects of disease will be accepted as its defining characteristic and in which the physician's role will be reduced to that of a technician who measures or a mechanic who repairs. On the other hand, if the challenge is to be confronted, then biomedicine must undergo a thorough and rigorous "rehumanization": the physician's role must be reconceived as one that effectively balances the scientific and the humanistic, and sick people, rather than their diseases, must once again be placed at the center of the medical enterprise—the center they now occupy only in these narratives of illness.

I want to end this study of pathography in its past and present forms with a glance toward possibilities for the future. What shapes will pathographies assume in the decades ahead? On the medical side, we can assume that such books will continue to reflect medical practice, whether this turns out to be a yet more refined and ultrascientific technology, replete with miracle drugs and genetic cures; or a more humane and patient-oriented medicine that emphasizes prevention no less than cure; or the impersonal and bureaucratic operation of large-scale public-health programs. On the literary side, we can hope that such books will explore with greater depth and subtlety the mysteries of suffering, renewal, and death, so central to the experience of illness. The pathographies I have discussed are mostly content to remain on the level of popular culture, but the fictional pathographies of Leo Tolstoy and Thomas Mann suggest what can be accomplished in this literary form. As Anatole Broyard observes, "A critical illness is one of our momentous experiences, yet I haven't seen a single nonfiction book that does it justice" (13). Pathography is a genre that awaits its masterworks.

Another question about the pathographies of the future is whether the genre will include narratives describing illness as it is experienced by the poor, the homeless, and the disadvantaged.[1] It is striking that in none of the pathographies I have discussed is the cost of the treatments the patients undergo so much as mentioned; few discuss limitations of insurance coverage or problems in obtaining medical care—even pathographies about AIDS. This suggests that books of this kind are written by the middle class or the affluent; for the most part, their authors seem educated and articulate. To date, then, pathography seems to be a middle-class or upper-middle-class genre, and this implies limitations both of sensibility and experience. We will not learn from these books what illness or its treatment means for the very poor or marginalized, those whose encounter with the medical profession takes place in clinics, emergency rooms, or overcrowded city hospitals—or does not take place at all. It is unlikely that such patients will write books. Here, then, is a field for case study and reportage, perhaps for some medical Studs Terkel, skilled in giving voice to those who in our society so often remain voiceless. We need to know what common myths of illness are shared by both rich and poor, how these myths are inflected by economic and class factors, and whether there are other myths or metaphors that spring up among the medically deprived.

Another voice we need to hear is that of the physician. This may seem a paradoxical statement at the end of a book that so insists on returning the patient to the medical enterprise and so often contrasts the patient's voice to that of medicine. But the "physician's voice" I am referring to is not Elliot Mishler's "voice of medicine," with its litany of blood gases, test results, statistical probabilities, and treatment choices—that highly stylized way of speaking and writing which, besides its practical function, serves to define the profession and perhaps to defend its members against the indignity, pain, and futility they confront every day—but the voice of the individual who is inevitably lost in that impersonal professional voice. In my current work at a tertiary care medical center, I have come to know exemplary physicians, exemplary because their medical gaze focuses simultaneously on the disease and on the person with the disease. These doctors are easily identified by their patients, their students, and their colleagues, though they are not always honored or rewarded by our medical system. We need to hear from them. Here, pathographies are not much help. The portrait of the physician in a pathography is most often negative; when the image is positive, it is usually that of a savior or superhero. Of course a patient cannot fully know the human individual who wears the long white physician's coat, just as a doctor cannot fully know the human individual in the anonymous hospital smock. But if physicians need to have a fuller sense of the persons for whose medical care they are responsible—especially in this era of transplants and genetic engineering, when we have come to believe that medicine is capable of just about any miracle—patients need to have a fuller sense of the individual who is their physician.

We have harrowing accounts of the hardships of medical training, anecdotal reminiscences of retired doctors, fictional and semifictional stories by doctor-writers, and the "clinical tales" of neurologists and psychiatrists—but these are not enough. We need more writing that conveys the inner reality of what it is to be a physician in today's technological medical system.[2] I hope that this study of pathography, with its avowed aim of restoring the patient's voice to the medical enterprise, might help to prompt autobiographies, treatment narratives, or personal essays that restore the doctor's voice as well—the ordinary flesh-and-blood physician whose autonomy is increasingly restricted by insurance companies, governmental bureaucracy, and the ever-present threat of lawsuits; whose emotional involvement with patients not only exacts its own cost but often conflicts with obligations to family and to self; and who occasionally (but inevitably) makes mistakes; yet who still manages to feel deeply for patients, who treasures the rich intimacy in knowing other human beings under conditions of suffering and fear, and who clearly, visibly, palpably enjoys being a doctor. Only when we hear *both* the doctor's and the patient's voice will we have a medicine that is truly human.

APPENDIX

✦

This is a partial listing, organized by disease, of the many pathographies that have been published in the past thirty years. It is intended to guide readers toward books they might want to read in full. Criteria for inclusion are narratives published recently, narratives of high literary quality or of unusual interest, or narratives that are unique in presenting a particular disease category or treatment. I have had to exclude a great many pathographies about cancer because these are so numerous.

Specific information about disease, author, and subject is indicated in brackets. I have in special instances included information about treatments when they are unusual or of special interest. If illness and treatment occur in a country other than the United States, this has been so indicated. The abbreviations in bold print are meant to help readers with the content and orientation of the pathographies included and to indicate organizing myths and metaphors.

Alt = describing the use of alternative medicine
Ang = dominated by a tone of anger
Christian/Judaism/Buddhism/Mormon = emphasizing a religious approach to illness
Inf = providing information about a particular illness, and treatment
Pt&Dr = written by a patient and a doctor
Phys = written by a physician about his or her own illness
SG = author finds a patient support group helpful
HM = organizing mythos is healthy-mindedness
Jour = organizing myth is the journey
Mil = organizing myth is military
Nat = organizing metaphor is drawn from nature
Reb = organizing myth is death and rebirth
Spo = organizing metaphor is sports

* = of unusual interest or especially well-written

All pathographies are about author's own experience unless otherwise indicated.

Pathographies are listed according to these categories:
AIDS
Cancer—breast
Cancer—other
Cardiovascular disease
Lupus
Neurological diseases—multiple sclerosis
Neurological diseases—other
Other illnesses
Collections of pathographies (1) about AIDS (2) about cancer (3) other

AIDS

Arterburn, Jerry. *How Will I Tell My Mother?* Nashville, Tenn.: Oliver-Nelson: 1988. [about self] **Christian**

Asistent, Niro Markoff, with Paul Duffy. *Why I Survive AIDS.* New York: Fireside/ Simon & Schuster, 1991. [female author, follower of Bhagwan Shree Rajneesh, writes about self, who survives, and male lover, who dies] **HM / Jour / SG**

Clark, J. Michael. *Diary of a Southern Queen: An HIV+ Vision Quest.* Dallas, Tex.: Monument Press, 1990. [about self and male lover] **HM**

Cox, Elizabeth. *Thanksgiving: An AIDS Journal.* New York: Harper & Row, 1990. [about husband's illness and assisted suicide] **Alt / HM**

Dreuilhe, Emmanuel. *Mortal Embrace: Living with AIDS.* Translated by Linda Coverdale. New York: Hill & Wang/Farrar, Straus & Giroux, 1988. [about male lover and self] **Ang / Mil**

Glaser, Elizabeth, and Laura Palmer. *In the Absence of Angels: A Hollywood Family's Courageous Story.* New York: G. P. Putnam, 1991. [about self (mother) & two children] **Alt / HM / Mil**

Hostetler, Helen M. *A Time to Love.* Scottdale, Pa: Herald Press, 1989. [about son] **Christian**

Melton, George R. *Beyond AIDS: A Journey into Healing.* Beverly Hills, Calif.: Brotherhood Press,1988. [about self and male lover] **Alt / HM / anti-Mil / Reb / SG**

*Monette, Paul. *Borrowed Time: An AIDS Memoir.* San Diego, Calif.: Harcourt Brace Jovanovich, 1988. Reprint. New York: Avon, 1990. [about male lover's illness and death] **Mil / anti-HM**

Mordaunt, John. *Facing Up to AIDS: As Told to John Masterson*. Dublin, Ireland: The O'Brien Press, Ltd., 1989. [AIDS & drug addiction; in Ireland] **Alt / HM / SG**

Nassaney, Louie, with Glenn Kolb. *I Am Not a Victim: One Man's Triumph over Fear and AIDS*. Santa Monica, Calif.: Hay House, Inc., 1990. [about self; Louise Hays approach] **Alt / HM / SG**

Owen, Bob. *Roger's Recovery from AIDS*. Malibu, Calif.: DAVAR, 1987. [written by a physician about a patient] **HM**

Peabody, Barbara. *The Screaming Room*. San Diego, Calif.: Oak Tree Publications, 1986. [about son's illness and death] **Mil**

Pearson, Carol Lynn. *Good-Bye, I Love You*. New York: Random House, 1986. [about husband's illness and death] **Alt / HM / Mormon**

Peavey, Fran. *A Shallow Pool of Time: An HIV+ Woman Grapples with the AIDS Epidemic*. Philadelphia, Pa.: New Society Publishers, 1990. [about self & others]

Perry, Shireen, with Gregg Lewis. *In Sickness and in Health: A Story of Love in the Shadow of AIDS*. Downers Grove, Ill.: Intervarsity Press, 1989. [about husband's illness and death] **Christian**

Reed, Paul. *The Q Journal*. Berkeley, Calif.: Celestial Arts, 1991. [author's experience with Compound Q (an unapproved experimental drug) and mourning for his male lover] **SG**

Rodale, Ardath H. *Climbing toward the Light*. Emmaus, Pa.: The Good Spirit Press, 1989. [about son's illness and death] **Christian**

Rozar, G. Edward, Jr., with David B. Biebel. *Laughing in the Face of AIDS: A Surgeon's Personal Battle*. Grand Rapids, Mich.: Baker Book House, 1992. [thoracic surgeon with AIDS] **Christian / Phys**

Tynes, Clairee. *The Miracle of Bill: A Family Confronts AIDS*. Cincinnati, Ohio: Forward Movement Publications, 1989. [about son's illness and death]

Cancer—Breast

Blumberg, Rena. *Headstrong: A Story of Conquests & Celebrations . . . Living Through Chemotherapy*. New York: Crown Publishers, Inc., 1982. **Alt / HM / Mil**

Brack, Pat, with Ben Brack. *Moms Don't Get Sick*. Melius Publishing Co., 1990. [focuses on how a parent's cancer experience affects their children] **HM / SG**

Brinker, Nancy, with Catherine McEvily Harris. *The Race Is Run One Step at a Time: My Personal Struggle—and Everywoman's Guide—to Taking Charge of Breast Cancer.* New York: Simon & Schuster, 1990. **Inf**

Britton, Janet. *To Live Each Moment: One Woman's Struggle against Cancer.* Downers Grove, Ill.: Intervarsity Press, 1984.

Butler, Sandra, and Barbara Rosenblum. *Cancer in Two Voices.* San Francisco, Calif.: Spinster Books, 1991. [illness and death of female lover] **HM / Judaism / SG**

Cler, Alice Elaine, and Barbara Cler Pendleton. *Cancer, God, and I, and a Natural Cure.* New York: Vantage, 1987. [naturopathic cure] **Alt / HM**

Comfort, Georgia, with Philip Comfort. *Dying to Live.* Wheaton, Ill.: Tyndale House Publishers Inc., 1992. [bone marrow transplant] **Christian**

Graham, Jory. *In the Company of Others.* New York: Harcourt Brace Jovanovich, 1982. **anti-HM / Inf**

Hargrove, Anne C. *Getting Better: Conversations with Myself and Other Friends While Healing from Breast Cancer.* Minneapolis, Minn.: CompCare Publishers, 1988. **HM / Reb**

Humphrey, Derek, with Ann Wickett. *Jean's Way.* New York: Quartet Books, 1978. Reprint. New York: Harper & Row/Perennial, 1986; Eugene, Oreg: Hemlock Society, 1991. [wife's illness and assisted suicide]

Hunsberger, Eydie Mae, and Chris Loeffler. *How I Conquered Cancer Naturally.* Garden City Park, N.Y.: Avery Publishing Group, Inc., 1992 [Ann Wigmore's Wheatgrass-therapy] **Alt**

Ireland, Jill. *Life Wish.* Boston, Mass.: Little, Brown and Co., 1987. **Alt / HM**

Johnson, Lois Walfred. *Either Way, I Win: A Guide for Growth in the Power of Prayer.* Minneapolis, Minn.: Augsburg Publishing House, 1979. **Christian**

*Lorde, Audre. *The Cancer Journals.* Argyle, N.Y.: Spinsters, 1980. Reprint. San Francisco: Spinsters Aunt Lute, 1987. **Mil / Reb**

Metzger, Deena. "Tree," in *The Woman Who Slept with Men and Tree.* Berkeley, Calif.: Wingbow Press, 1978; 1981. **Mil**

Mitchell, Joyce Slayton. *Winning the Chemo Battle.* New York: W. W. Norton, 1988. **Inf / Mil**

Photopulos, Georgia and Bud. *Of Tears and Triumphs.* New York: Congdon and Weed, Inc., 1988. [an account of unusually aggressive treatments]

Rollin, Betty. *First, You Cry.* Philadelphia, Pa.: J. B. Lippincott, 1976.

Schwerin, Doris. *Diary of a Pigeon Watcher.* New York: William Morrow & Co., 1976. **Nat / anti-Reb**

*Shapero, Lucy, and Anthony A. Goodman. *Never Say Die: A Doctor and a Patient Talk about Breast Cancer.* New York: Appleton, 1980. **HM / Pt&Dr**

Snyder, Marilyn. *An Informed Decision: Understanding Breast Reconstruction.* New York: M. Evans & Co., 1984. [about self and others] **Inf**

Wallin, Bernice, with Fred Wallin. *I Beat Cancer.* Chicago, Ill: Contemporary Books, Inc., 1978. [describing an experimental research treatment (BCG)] **Alt / HM**

Wecksler, Becky Lynn & Michael. *In God's Hand: One Woman's Experience with Breast Cancer.* Scottdale, Pa.: Herald Press, 1989. **Christian / HM**

Wilber, Ken. *Grace and Grit: Spirituality and Healing in the Life and Death of Treya Killam Wilber.* Boston, Mass.: Shambhala, 1991. [wife's illness and death] **Alt / HM / New Age Buddhist / SG**

Cancer—Other

Anderson, Greg. *The Cancer Conquerer: An Incredible Journey to Wellness.* Kansas City, Mo.: Andrews and McMeel, 1988. Reprint. 1990; 1992. [lung cancer] **HM / Mil**

*Beauvoir, Simone de. *A Very Easy Death.* Translated by Patrick O'Brien. New York: G. P. Putnam, 1965. Reprint. New York: Pantheon, 1985. [mother's pancreatic cancer and death; in France]

Bedsworth, Philip and Joyce. *Fight the Good Fight.* Scottdale, Pa.: Herald Press, 1991. [chronic myelogenous leukemia; bone marrow transplant] **Christian / Mil**

Benedict, Dirk. *Confessions of a Kamikaze Cowboy.* North Hollywood, Calif.: Newcastle Publishing Co., 1987. [prostate cancer; macrobiotics] **Alt / Ang**

Berté, Raymond A. *To Speak Again: Victory over Cancer.* Agawam, Mass.: Phillips Publishing Company, 1987. [throat cancer; Bernie Siegel approach] **Alt / HM**

Bishop, Beata. *My Triumph over Cancer: The Therapy of the Future.* New Canaan, Conn.: Keats Publishing Co., 1986. [melanoma; Gerson therapy; in England] **Alt / HM**

*Broyard, Anatole. *Intoxicated by My Illness and Other Writings on Life and Death.* Edited by Alexandra Broyard. New York: Clarkson Potter, 1992. [Broyard's prostate cancer; also father's bladder cancer and death]

Conley, Herbert N. *Living and Dying Gracefully.* New York: Paulist Press, 1979. [colon cancer; about Christian dying] **Inf / Christian**

Cook, Stephanie. *Second Life.* New York: Simon & Schuster, 1981. [choriocarcinoma] **Ang / anti-Reb**

Craig, Jean. *Between Hello & Goodbye: A Life-Affirming Story of Courage in the Face of Tragedy.* Los Angeles, Calif.: Jeremy P. Tarcher, Inc., 1991. [husband's colon cancer and death; describing an experimental research protocol] **Ang / Mil**

*Creaturo, Barbara. *Courage: The Testimony of a Cancer Patient.* New York: Pantheon, 1991. [ovarian cancer; describing an experimental treatment] **anti-HM / Mil**

Dravecky, Dave, with Tim Stafford. *Comeback.* Grand Rapids, Mich.: Zondervan Publishing House; San Francisco, Calif: Harper and Row, 1990. [tumor of the deltoid muscle] **Spo**

Dravecky, Dave & Jan, with Ken Gire. *When You Can't Come Back.* Grand Rapids, Mich.: Zondervan Publishing House; San Francisco, Calif.: Harper/San Francisco, 1992. [metastatic desmoid tumor; amputation] **Christian**

Epstein, Alice Hopper. *Mind, Fantasy and Healing: One Woman's Journey from Conflict and Illness to Wholeness and Health.* New York: Delacorte; Bantam, 1989. [kidney cancer] **Alt / HM / Mil**

Farnsworth, Ken. *Journey to Healing.* St. Louis, Mo.: The Christian Board of Publications, 1985. [leimyosarcoma of the vena cava] **Christian**

Fiore, Neil A. *The Road Back to Health: Coping with the Emotional Side of Cancer.* Toronto: Bantam, 1984. [testicular cancer] **Alt / HM**

*Frank, Arthur W. *At the Will of the Body: Reflections on Illness.* Boston, Mass.: Houghton Mifflin, 1991. [testicular cancer; also heart attack; in Canada] **anti-Mil**

Geier, Mary Alice. *Cancer, What's It Doing in My Life?* Pasadena, Calif.: Hope Publishing House, 1985. [progressive lymphoma; about living with the effects of chemotherapy] **HM / anti-Mil / SG**

Helman, Ethel. *An Autumn Life: How a Surgeon Faced His Fatal Illness.* London: Faber & Faber, 1986. [constructed from husband-surgeon's tapes about his own colon cancer; also her account of his death] **Ang / Phys**

Hine, Virginia. *Last Letter to the Pebble People: "Aldie Soars."* Santa Cruz, Calif.: Unity Press, 1977. [husband's lung cancer and death] Alt / HM

Hingle, Patricia. *A Coming of Roses.* Prairieville, La.: Home Plates of Ascension, Inc., 1988. [squamous cell carcinoma of the neck] **Nat / Reb**

Howe, Herbert. *Do Not Go Gentle.* New York: Norton, 1981. [fibrosarcoma of the wrist] **HM / Spo**

*Lerner, Gerda. *A Death of One's Own.* New York: Simon & Schuster, 1978. [husband's inoperable brain cancer and assisted suicide]

Lerner, Max. *Wrestling with the Angel: A Memoir of My Triumph over Illness.* New York: W. W. Norton, 1990. [large cell lymphoma and prostate cancer; also heart attack] **HM**

Malcolm, Andrew. *Someday.* New York: Knopf, 1991. [mother's lung cancer and death]

Meryman, Richard. *Hope: A Loss Survived.* Boston, Mass.: Little, Brown & Co., 1980. [wife's melanoma and death]

Mullan, Fitzhugh. *Vital Signs: A Young Doctor's Struggle with Cancer.* New York: Farrar, Straus, Giroux, 1975. [pediatrician with testicular cancer] **Phys / anti-Reb**

*Noll, Peter. *In the Face of Death.* Translated by Hans Noll. New York: Viking/Penguin, 1989. [bladder cancer and death; commentary on facing death]

Nussbaum, Elaine. *Recovery from Cancer to Health through Macrobiotics.* Tokyo & New York: Japan Publications, Inc., 1986. [endometrial cancer; macrobiotics] **Alt**

O'Connell, Anne. *First Cancer Then Lupus: The Courageous Story of One Woman's Journey through Illness, Chemotherapy, Steroids, and Pain Control.* San Diego, Calif.: Custom Books, 1991. [lymphoma, and lupus] **HM**

Oden, Rev. Clifford. *Thank God I Have Cancer!* New Rochelle, N.Y.: Arlington House, 1976. [colon cancer; laetrile] **Alt / Christian**

Priest, Mary Woodward. *Diary of Courage: Coping with Life-threatening Illness.* San Francisco, Calif.: Strawberry Hill Press, 1990. [husband's prostate cancer] **Inf**

*Radner, Gilda. *It's Always Something.* New York: Simon & Schuster, 1989. Reprint. New York: Avon, 1990. [ovarian cancer] **Alt / HM / Mil / SG**

Rodman, Robert F. *Not Dying.* New York: Random House, 1977. [wife's ovarian/gastrointestinal cancer and death; in Sweden] **Alt**

Rollin, Betty. *Last Wish*. New York: Warner Books, 1985. [mother's ovarian cancer and assisted suicide]

Rosenbaum, Edward E. *A Taste of My Own Medicine: When the Doctor Is the Patient*. New York: Random House, 1988; reprinted as *The Doctor: When the Doctor Is the Patient*. [rheumatologist with cancer of vocal cord] **Ang / Phys**

*Roth, Philip. *Patrimony: A True Story*. New York: Simon & Schuster, 1991. [father's brain tumor; also author's own emergency quintuple bypass surgery]

*Ryan, Cornelius, and Kathryn Morgan. *A Private Battle*. New York: Fawcett, 1979. [prostate cancer] **Mil**

Sanes, Samuel. *A Physician Faces Cancer in Himself*. Albany: State University of New York Press, 1979. [pathologist with reticulum cell sarcoma; on the need for doctors to better communicate with their patients] **Mil / Phys**

*Sattilaro, Anthony J., with Tom Monte. *Recalled by Life: The Story of My Recovery from Cancer*. Boston, Mass.: Houghton Mifflin, 1982. [anaesthesiologist with prostate cancer; macrobiotics] **Alt / HM / Phys**

Schreiber, LeAnne. *Midstream*. New York: Viking Penguin, 1990. [mother's pancreatic cancer and death] **Nat**

Shapiro, Kenneth A. *Dying and Living: One Man's Life with Cancer*. Austin: University of Texas Press, 1985. [melanoma] **HM / Mil**

Snow, Lois Wheeler. *A Death with Dignity: When the Chinese Came*. New York: Random House, 1974. [husband's pancreatic cancer and death; in Switzerland; Chinese medical care] **Alt**

Soiffer, Bill. *Life in the Shadow: Living with Cancer*. San Francisco, Calif.: Chronicle Books, 1991. [Hodgkin's disease] **anti-HM / Inf / Mil**

Tate, David A. *Health, Hope, and Healing*. New York: M. Evans & Company, 1989. [Hodgkin's disease; also heart attack] **Alt / Reb**

Thompson, Francesca Morosani. *Going for the Cure*. New York: St. Martin's, 1989. [orthopaedic surgeon with multiple myeloma] **HM / Phys**

Ulrich, Betty Garton. *Rooted in the Sky: A Faith to Cope with Cancer*. Valley Forge, Pa.: Judson Press, 1989. [colon cancer] **Christian**

Wertenbaker, Lael Tucker. *Death of a Man*. New York: Random House, 1957. [husband's intestinal cancer and assisted suicide]

Widome, Allen. *The Doctor/The Patient: The Personal Journey of a Physician with Cancer.* Miami, Fla.: Editech Press, 1989. [anesthesiologist with non-Hodgkin's lymphoma] **Phys / Ang**

*Williams, Terry Tempest. *Refuge: An Unnatural History of Family and Place.* New York: Pantheon, 1991. [mother's ovarian cancer and death] **anti-Mil / Mormon / Nat**

Cardiovascular Disease

Barbree, Jay. *The Day I Died: One Man's Successful Battle Back from the Dead.* Far Hills, N.J.: New Horizon Press, 1990. [cardiac arrest and bypass surgery] **Reb**

Brown, H.C., Jr. *Walking toward Your Fear.* Nashville, Tenn.: Broadman, 1972. [mitral and aortic valve replacement surgery] **Jour**

Castelli, Jim. *I'm Too Young to Have a Heart Attack.* Rochlin, Calif.: Prime Publishing Co., 1990. [MI (heart attack)] **HM**

Cousins, Norman. *The Healing Heart: Antidotes to Panic and Helplessness.* New York: Norton, 1983. [heart muscle destruction and congestive heart failure] **HM**

Halberstam, Michael, and Stephan Lesher. *A Coronary Event.* New York: Popular Library; CBS Publications, 1978. [MI] **Pt&Dr**

Johnson, James L. *Coming Back: One Man's Journey to the Edge of Eternity and Spiritual Rediscovery.* Springhouse, 1979. [angina; four-vessel coronary bypass surgery] **Christian / Jour / Reb**

King, Larry, with B. D. Colen. *"Mr. King, You're Having a Heart Attack."* New York: Bantam; Doubleday, 1989. [MI; bypass surgery]

*Lear, Martha Weinman. *Heartsounds: The Story of a Love and Loss.* New York: Simon & Schuster, 1980. [urologist-husband's MI, bypass surgery and removal of aneurysm in left ventricle, post-op brain damage] **Ang / Mil / Phys**

Mandell, Arnold J. *Coming of Middle Age: A Journey.* New York: Summit, 1977. [threatened MI and coronary artery disease] **Jour / Phys / Reb**

Nolan, William A. *Surgeon under the Knife.* New York: Coward, McCann & Geoghegan Inc., 1976. [surgeon with coronary artery disease; bypass surgery] **Inf / Phys**

Reinfeld, Nyles V. *Open Heart Surgery: A Second Chance.* Englewood Cliffs, N.J.: Prentice-Hall, Inc., 1983. [bypass surgery] **Pt&Dr / Inf / Reb**

See also Frank, Lerner, Roth, and Tate under "Cancer—Other."

Lupus

Aladjem, Henrietta, and Peter H. Schur. *In Search of the Sun: A Woman's Courageous Victory over Lupus*. New York: MacMillan, 1988. **Inf / Pt&Dr**

Brown, Beverly D. *I Choose to Live!* Nashville, Tenn.: Winston-Derek Publishers, Inc., 1990. **SG**

Chester, Laura. *Lupus Novice: Toward Self-Healing*. Barrytown, N.Y.: Station Hill Press, 1987. **Alt / HM**

Permut, Joanna Baumer. *Embracing the Wolf: A Lupus Victim and Her Family Learn to Live with Chronic Disease*. Atlanta, Ga: Cherokee Publishing Co., 1989.

Radziunas, Eileen. *Lupus: My Search for a Diagnosis*. Edited by Jackie Melvin. Claremont, Calif.: Hunter House, 1989. **Ang**

Szasz, Susy. *Living with It: Why You Don't Have to Be Healthy to Be Happy*. Buffalo, N.Y.: Prometheus Books, 1991. **Inf**

See also O'Connell under "Cancer."

Neurological Diseases: Multiple Sclerosis

Atwood, Dave. *Tomorrow is a Better Day*. New York: Vantage, 1986.

Breslow, Rachelle. *Who Said So? A Woman's Journey of Self Discovery and Triumph over Multiple Sclerosis*. Berkeley, Calif.: Celestial Arts, 1991. **Alt**

Michael, Peter Paul. *Multiple Sclerosis: A Dragon with a Hundred Heads*. Port Washington, N.Y.: Ashley Books, Inc., 1981. [experimental regimen involving ACTH] **Christian**

*Webster, Barbara D. *All of a Piece: A Life with Multiple Sclerosis*. Baltimore, Md.: Johns Hopkins University Press, 1989. **anti-HM**

Neurological Diseases: Other

Atwood, Glenna Wotton, with Lila Green Hunnewell. *Living Well with Parkinson's*. New York: John Wiley & Sons, 1991. [Parkinsonism] **Inf**

Baier, Sue, and Mary Zimmeth. *Bed Number Ten*. New York: Holt Rinehart & Winston, 1986. [Guillain-Barré syndrome] **Ang**

Davidson, Andrea L. *Embrace the Dawn: One Woman's Story of Triumph over Epilepsy*. McCall, Idaho: Sylvan Creek Press, 1989. [epilepsy with temporal lobectomy, post-op depression]

Fishman, Steve. *A Bomb in the Brain: A Heroic Tale of Science, Surgery, and Survival.* New York: Charles Scribner's Sons, 1988. [brain hemorrhage & surgery; epilepsy] **Inf**

Jones, Terry L., with David F. Nixon. *Venom in My Veins: One Man's Battle against Lou Gehrig's Disease.* Kansas City, Mo.: Beacon Hill Press, 1985. [amyotrophic lateral sclerosis; experimental regimen involving injections of cobra venom] **Christian**

Kovek, Carol Wolfe. *Daddyboy: A Memoir.* St. Paul, Minn.: Graywolf Press, 1991. [father's Alzheimer's disease and death from pneumonia]

Malcolm, Andrew H. *This Far and No More: A True Story.* New York: Times Books/Random House, 1987. [author uses Emily Bauer's diary entries to write about her amyotrophic lateral sclerosis and death by assisted suicide]

Mille, Agnes de. *Reprieve: A Memoir.* New York: Doubleday,1981. [stroke] **Reb**

*Murphy, Robert. *The Body Silent.* New York: Henry Holt & Co., 1987. [spinal cord disease; quadraplegia] **Jour**

Reese, Robert. *Healing Fits: The Curing of an Epileptic.* Los Angeles, Calif.: Big Sky Press, 1988. [epilepsy (pseudo-epilepsy?); Primal Therapy] **Alt / HM**

Sarton, May. *After the Stroke: A Journal.* New York: Norton, 1988. [stroke] **Reb**

Severo, Richard. *Lisa H.: The True Story of an Extraordinary and Courageous Woman.* New York: Harper & Row, 1985. [facial neurofibromatosis]

Shirk, Evelyn. *After the Stroke: Coping with America's Third Leading Cause of Death.* Buffalo, N.Y.: Prometheus Books, 1991. [husband's experience with a series of strokes] **Inf**

Simpson, Elizabeth Leone. *Notes on an Emergency: A Journal of Recovery.* New York: W. W. Norton & Co., 1982. [tubercular meningitis; coma] **HM**

Vaughan, Ivan. *Ivan: Living with Parkinson's Disease.* New York: Farrar, Straus, Giroux, 1986. [Parkinsonism in 40-year-old man] **Alt / HM**

Other Illnesses

Blakely, Mary Kay. *Wake Me When It's Over: A Journey to the Edge and Back.* New York: Times Books, 1989. [diabetes & sarcoidosis, coma] **HM / Reb**

Bradley, Denise J. *What Does It Feel Like to Have Diabetes: A Diary of Events in the Life of a Diabetic.* Springfield, Ill.: Charles C. Thomas, 1987. [diabetes] **HM**

Clark, Eleanor. *Eyes, Etc.: A Memoir.* New York: Pantheon, 1977. [macular degeneration] **Ang**

*Cousins, Norman. *Anatomy of an Illness As Perceived by the Patient: Reflections on Healing and Regeneration.* New York: Norton, 1979. [ankylosing spondylitis] **HM**

Goshen-Gottstein, Esther. *Recalled to Life: The Story of a Coma.* New Haven, Conn.: Yale University Press, 1990. [coma following bypass surgery] **Jour**

Greene, Mary Cooper. *Living with a Broken String.* Springboro, Pa.: Greene Associates, 1987. [diabetes] **Christian**

Maier, Frank & Ginny. *Sweet Reprieve: One Couple's Journey to the Frontiers of Medicine.* New York: Crown Publisher Inc., 1991. [chronic active hepatitis; liver transplant] **Inf / Jour / Reb**

*Sacks, Oliver. *A Leg to Stand On.* New York: Summit Books, 1984. [neurologist with leg injury] **Ang / Jour / Phys**

Collections: AIDS

Callen, Michael. *Surviving AIDS.* New York: Harper Perennial/ HarperCollins, 1990. [stories of long-term survivors, mostly homosexual] **Alt / HM / SG**

Gregory, Scott J., and Bianca Leonardo. *They Conquered AIDS: True Life Adventures from Self-Reliance, through Inspiration, into Transformation.* Palm Springs, Calif.: Tree of Life Publications, 1989. **Alt / HM / SG**

Hitchens, Neal. *Voices That Care: Stories and Encouragement for People with AIDS/HIV and Those Who Love Them.* Los Angeles, Calif.: Lowell House, 1992. [brief pathographies of men, women, and children] **Alt / HM / SG**

Petrow, Steven. *Dancing against the Darkness: A Journey through America in the Age of AIDS.* Lexington, Mass.: D. C. Heath and Co., 1990. [pathographies of a wide variety of people with AIDS]

Rider, Ines, and Patricia Ruppelt, eds. *AIDS: The Women.* San Francisco: Cleis, 1988.

Rudd, Andrea, and Darien Taylor. *Positive Women: Views of Women Living with AIDS.* Toronto: Second Story Press, 1992. [38 pathographies from women all over the world who are HIV+ or have AIDS] **SG**

Tilleraas, Perry. *Circle of Hope: Our Stories of AIDS, Addictions, and Recovery.* NP: Hazelden, 1990. [AIDS combined with drug and/or alcohol addiction] **SG**

Collections: Cancer

Fay, Martha. *A Mortal Condition: Eight Portraits of Survival, Loss, and Hope.* New York: Coward-McCann, Inc., 1983. [eight cancer patients at Memorial Sloan-Kettering]

*Glassman, Judith. *The Cancer Survivors and How They Did It.* New York: The Dial Press; Doubleday & Company, 1983. [long-term cancer survivors and the treatments used—especially those involving alternative therapies] **Alt / HM**

Kahane, Deborah H. *No Less a Woman: Ten Women Shatter the Myths about Breast Cancer.* New York: Prentice Hall Press; Simon & Schuster, 1990. [focus is on psychological recovery, especially how to keep self-esteem intact]

Moss, Ralph W. *A Real Choice.* New York: St. Martin's, 1984. [seven women with breast cancer; detection and treatment options]

Pepper, Curtis Bill. *We the Victors: Inspiring Stories of People Who Conquered Cancer and How They Did It.* Garden City, N.Y.: Doubleday and Co., Inc., 1984. [five factors important to survive: love, self, need, luck, the best (orthodox) treatment]

Shook, Robert L. *Survivors: Living with Cancer, Portraits of Twelve Inspiring People.* New York: Harper and Row, 1983. [survivors via orthodox cancer treatment]

*Williams, Wendy. *The Power Within: True Stories of Exceptional Patients Who Fought Back with Hope.* New York: Harper and Row, 1990. [ten cancer patients who benefited from alternative therapies and cancer support groups] **Alt / HM / SG**

Collections: Other

Mandell, Harvey, and Howard Spiro. *When Doctors Get Sick.* New York and London: Plenum Medical Book Co., 1987. [a variety of illnesses] **Phys**

Preface

1. It is true that some diseases, such as prostate cancer or ovarian cancer, are gender specific. Breast cancer can afflict men, but its significance for a woman is obviously different, and all the pathographies I have read about this illness are by (or about) women. As my Appendix shows, a great many patients deal with breast cancer and its treatment by writing about it: an unusual number of pathographies fall in this category. Moreover, some strategies for coping with illness and treatment seem to be gender specific. Pathographies demonstrate that women and homosexual men tend to use patient support-groups far more frequently than do heterosexual men. My Appendix shows that all instances when an author mentions the helpfulness of a support group are pathographies written by women or homosexual men. Aside from these two examples, I have found little evidence that differences in pathography can be attributed to the sexual identity of the author. For example, conventional stereotyping might lead us to expect that the myth of battle would appeal especially to males, but in fact it appears as an organizing myth in pathographies by authors of both sexes. It is of course possible to make gender an overt and important issue in one's formulation. This is what Audre Lorde does in her splendid *The Cancer Journals.* Lorde writes as a woman, but as a woman who is "a black lesbian feminist" (24–25). This identity is central to her formulation and explains her conviction that giving voice to certain important personal experiences is by nature a political gesture: to remain silent about one's breast cancer or mastectomy not only denies oneself the support of other women but also relegates that experience to "the tyrannies of silence" (20).

Chapter 1: *Introduction*

1. I first encountered the term "pathography" when reading Oliver Sacks's *Awakenings,* where the word is used to refer to biographies that combine science and art—"the most perfect examples" of which are "the matchless case-histories of Freud" (1990, 229). It must be observed that in the 1990 edition of *Awakenings,* Sacks adds a few sentences to a footnote (on the same page) where he again uses the term "pathography," though this time with rather a different meaning. Here the term is used pejoratively to refer to case histories that are "histories of disease" rather than "histories of people, histories of *life*" (229–30). In the 1983 Dutton paperback edition of *Awakenings,* the word

"pathography" seems to have been misprinted as "pathology" (206). Freud uses the word "pathography" in *Leonardo Da Vinci and a Memory of His Childhood* (the term may well appear in other of his writings as well). Pathography here refers to a biographical study that focuses on the way pathological elements in a person's life can illumine other facets of that life. Thus, Freud calls his study of Leonardo a pathography, observing that "the aim of our work has been to explain the inhibitions in Leonardo's sexual life and in his artistic activity" (81). I use "pathography" to refer to an autobiographical or biographical narrative about an experience of illness.

2. *Culture* is a tricky word. At one extreme, we use the term *Western culture* to refer to the heritage of ideas and conventions derived from classical and Judaeo-Christian sources. At the other, we perceive different racial, national, religious, or economic groups as constituting different cultures or perhaps subcultures of a given society. I will be using the term to refer to a gestalt of attitudes, practices, conventions, and expectations held in common by a majority of people living in a given national region or regions. Since most of my pathographies are written and published in the United States, and since, as a U.S. citizen, I am most familiar with my own country's conventions and ideas about illness, the culture I refer to is, broadly speaking, American. The attitudes toward illness in other Western nations where scientific medicine is the predominant health-care system will quite probably be very similar to those I call American; however, Lynn Payer's *Medicine and Culture,* a fine study that documents subtle differences in ideas about illness and treatment characteristic of Germany, France, Great Britain, and the United States, teaches me to be careful in assuming anything more than a similarity.

The pathographies upon which I base my study are culled from those written in or translated into English. I feel I can treat Simone de Beauvoir's *A Very Easy Death* as a pathography representative of American attitudes because its popularity in translation suggests a resonance with its American readers.

The authors of pathographies are for the most part middle-class patients; most often U.S. citizens. But the readership of these books may well be a good deal broader than the authorship: it would therefore be inaccurate to claim that the myths and attitudes about illness that can be found in these books are exclusively restricted to middle-class Americans. We do know, given the increasing numbers of pathographies in print each year, that there are a great many potential readers for these books, and thus there is justification in claiming that the myths about illness in pathographies are representative of a fairly large segment of the population.

Despite the fact that illness in the United States is most often treated in accord with the same medical model, it is important that one not assume a similarity in the medical experience of patients from all classes and different racial backgrounds. Even given a broad allowance for an unknowable readership, it must be recognized that pathographies probably do not represent the way illness is experienced by the poor. A collection of pathographies gathered from the indigent and the homeless or from racial minorities (a project I hope to undertake) might well reflect a very different set of cultural myths about illness. Readers interested in this first group will want to look at Michael A. Susko's *Cry of the Invisible,* a collection of autobiographical poems and prose pieces by homeless persons and by survivors of mental hospitals; those with an interest in the illness experience of racial minorities will want to look at Marian Gray Secundy's *Trials, Tribulations, and Celebrations,* a collection of fictional and autobiographical pieces by African-Americans, and Barbara Blair and Susan E. Cayliff's *Wings of Gauze: Women of Color and the Experience of Health and Illness.*

3. The pathographies of physicians who describe their own illness experience could themselves be the subject of a separate study. I include several such pathographies in *Reconstructing Illness* but do not consider them in the text as a separate category. A fine collection of these narratives, *When Doctors Get Sick,* has been compiled by Harvey Mandell and Howard Spiro. See also the books by physician-authors noted in the Appendix.

4. Kathryn Montgomery Hunter, in *Doctor Stories: The Narrative Structure of Medical Knowledge,* includes a helpful discussion of the differences between the patient's (oral) story of illness and the physician's narrative (62–63) and between pathography and case history (154–55). Since this book appeared after I had completed *Reconstructing Illness,* I was not able to take advantage of Hunter's admirable commentary on medical narrative.

5. The problem with Kleinman's notion, however, is that the patient's explanatory model must be both constructed and interpreted by the physician: "the clinician must first piece together the illness narrative as it emerges from the patient's and the family's complaints and explanatory models; then he or she must interpret it" (49). The patient, then, only "speaks" through the physician's capacity to listen, understand, and interpret. Kleinman does not discuss the problems inherent in such a formula.

6. This movement toward the social element in autobiography—its "extrospective" dimensions—has been helped along by critics writing about the function of autobiography for minorities and for women. The existence of the self is never really an issue here; instead, autobiographical documents are seen as invaluable in recovering lost or marginal social and cultural dimensions of human existence.

7. Kleinman uses the word *myth* in writing about a patient's explanatory model, referring to "the sick individual's personal myth [as] a story that gives shape to an illness" (49). His sense of the mythic seems to me somewhat limited

in that it is restricted to self-deception: "Myth making, a universal human quality, reassures us that resources conform to our desires rather than to actual descriptions. In short, self-deception makes chronic illness tolerable" (48).

8. Robert Segal's fine essay, "In Defense of Mythology: the History of Modern Theories of Myth," a succinct and intelligent summary of modern theories of myth beginning with Tylor, is one of the best I have read on the subject. I am indebted to Segal for alerting me to the importance of Bultmann in the history of myth criticism.

9. The end result of Bultmann's "demythologizing" the New Testament, unlike its nineteenth-century counterpart, is to affirm the truth of New Testament kerygma. Bultmann criticizes nineteenth-century demythologizing for eliminating the kerygma along with the mythology and recent attempts at "repristinating New Testament mythology" for "making the kerygma unintelligible for the present" (11). Bultmann's approach is remarkably close to medieval allegory: the literal meaning of the New Testament is here considered a dispensable "shell" for the kerygma, the kernel of truth within.

10. David Barnard has alerted me to the fact that in actual practice many patients have themselves internalized the mechanistic metaphor, using it to ward off the *physician's* attempts to direct the patient's attention to social or emotional issues in illness. An example of this is the patient who somatizes. This kind of behavior, however, is rarely represented in pathography.

11. This section on Sontag and metaphoric thinking is based on a talk I gave in 1986 at a MLA special session on Literature and Medicine chaired by Anne Hudson Jones. Albert Howard Carter III, in his essay "Metaphors in the Physician-Patient Relationship," makes a similar argument. Carter goes on to discuss ways in which metaphoric language facilitates communication between doctor and patient.

12. The first two elements in Lifton's idea of formulation, the sense of connection and the sense of symbolic integrity, are very similar to two of the three elements I have identified as essential to any functional myth: that it be integrative, bringing together experience into a unified whole; and that it be connective, relating the individual experience to some larger whole.

13. Lifton finds that survivors whose formulative process is impaired often carry with them an "indelible image" of the experience—an image that prevents the individual from ever moving beyond the traumatic experience: "One remains fixed upon the world that has been annihilated, held motionless because unable to give form to that annihilation and its consequences" (1967, 528). In pathography, instead of the "indelible image" that impairs formulation for Lifton's Hiroshima survivors, one often finds a "mythic image" that enhances formulation.

Chapter 2: *The Myth of Rebirth and the Promise of Cure*

1. The kind of broad cultural contrast I have drawn here inevitably simplifies and exaggerates. I do not mean to imply that religion is *not* an important and pervasive element in our present culture; I am also aware that, in recent decades, there may have been an increase in religious interest and commitment. But religion today is not a central and controlling force affecting every facet of cultural life, as it clearly was in seventeenth-century England. My point is that this difference is reflected in writings about illness.

2. See Hawkins, *Archetypes of Conversion,* for an extended discussion of conversion in spiritual autobiography.

3. It is worth noting that for a surprising number of converts (Augustine, for example, and quite possibly Paul), physical illness is the occasion of the author's conversion. This is true of Ken Farnsworth's experience as he describes it in *The Ultimate Healing.* Farnsworth wakes up from surgery for removal of a huge tumor from his inferior vena cava to hear his surgeon tell him that he "got all the tumor": "It was at that point I knew I was healed of cancer. It was also at that very moment that I knew I was converted. That moment remains my time of conversion" (5).

4. See Bill Cowie, "The Cardiac Patient's Perception of His Heart Attack."

5. Roger Sharrock, in *John Bunyan,* 59, is quoting "To Mrs. St. John," I, *Letters and Speeches of Oliver Cromwell,* ed. Thomas Carlyle, 51–52.

6. Mandell's unusual comparison of personality to neuroscience's construct of the triadic brain betrays the author's skepticism about the possibility of change even as it validates it: "Changing [character] without major neurobiological alteration," he observes, "may be fantasy" (75).

7. In *The Type C Connection,* Lydia Temoshok and Henry Dreher explore the links between "type C behavior" (they carefully avoid the term "type C personality") and cancer. Pathographers tend to use the term "cancer-prone personality" more frequently than "type C personality"; indeed, the term "type C behavior" is almost never used.

8. For example, Jory Graham writes critically of the myth associating cancer with sin: "The idea that cancer is punishment for sin . . . [is] a solid belief. . . . most Americans believe, consciously or unconsciously, that cancer strikes as direct retribution for transgression, and that it must be suffered" (79). The only pathographies I have read that focus on the negative aspects of associating cancer with a certain personality type are Graham's, Sontag's, and Bill Soiffer's *Life in the Shadow: Living with Cancer.* It may be significant that though Graham's and Sontag's books are pathographies, and thus in some way are related to the author's need to come to terms with her own cancer experience, both narratives focus not so much on the author's personal experience of illness as on

general reflections about cancer. Graham's perspective is that of an informed cancer patient, offering insights on such issues as the choices patients have in their treatments, their right to know the facts about diagnosis and prognosis, and the right to be free of pain; Sontag's is that of an intellectual and an academic, researching the myths about cancer and tuberculosis found in literature. Soiffer's book interweaves his personal story of Hodgkin's disease with the stories of other such patients, and with the larger story of how medical science found a cure for this particular kind of cancer.

9. Carolyn Horsam, Nancy Reeves, Felicia Ackerman, "Letters to the Editor," *New York Times Magazine,* 3 Dec. 1989. At almost the same time the *New York Times Book Review* printed a similar series—a review article of a book, Jill Krementz's *How It Feels to Fight for Your Life,* and a letter criticizing the review for being part of "the trend of using selected people as models to 'inspire and instruct'" others in treating illness as "opportunities for personal growth and a deeper appreciation of life" (Review by Edwin Kenney, Jr., 12 Nov. 1989; letters, 24 Dec. 1989, again by Felicia Ackerman, and 14 Jan. 1990, by Kenney, rebutting Ackerman).

10. With two exceptions, Sandra Butler and Barbara Rosenblum's impressive *Cancer in Two Voices* and Ken Wilber's *Grace and Grit,* every pathography I have read that explicitly uses religion as the basis for its formulation is written by a Christian. Thus I discuss only Christianity as providing a religious frame of reference for pathography. In *Cancer in Two Voices,* Barbara Rosenblum, dying of metastatic breast cancer, turns to the rituals of Orthodox Judaism near the end of her life to give meaning to her experience. In *Grace and Grit,* Treya Wilber supplements both orthodox and alternative medical therapies for metastatic breast cancer with Buddhist meditations and teachings as well as inspirational lessons from transpersonal psychology and its "perennial philosophy."

11. Dravecky's second pathography—the story of his wife's depression, the return of his cancer and amputation of his arm, and the struggle both face in dealing not only with Dave's forced retirement from baseball but also with the instant fame that results from the astonishing success of *Comeback*—is a deeply religious book. We cannot fail to be moved by the fact that he prays for the surgical team in the operating room just before he has his arm amputated and by his brave attempts to respond to the question raised by so many of those who write to him: "Why does God make us suffer?" (120–21, 137–53). But the childlike faith this couple sustain throughout their ordeal ("Jan and I believed in a heavenly Father with big, strong hands that could fix anything" [25]) is brutally challenged by those Christians who claim to be trying to help them. For example, Jan is rebuked for seeking counseling for severe depression by both her pastor and the pastor's wife, who claim that all she needs is God and His Word (61–63); Dave is repeatedly advised by Christian well-wishers that

he would be cured of his cancer if his faith were strong enough (70, 72, 112–13). Paradoxically, the Draveckys are most helped with their nonmedical problems by their doctor—a sympathetic and compassionate man who recognizes that healing involves more than treating disease. Dr. McGowen not only diagnoses and treats Jan's mitral valve prolapse but also helps her recognize the connection between her cardiac irregularity, the stress she is experiencing, and her depression (65–68). Later on, when Dravecky comes to this same doctor with a peptic ulcer, he confides in him about his depression, his feeling about cancer recurring, and his fear of death. Dr. McGowen again succeeds—where Christian "advisors" in this pathography fail—in responding with charity and kindness: "It was normal to grieve, he told me, not a lack of faith. . . . One by one, Dr. McGowen addressed the problems I was having" (166).

12. Similarly, Donne's contemporary, the Anglican divine Jeremy Taylor, in *The Rule and Exercises of Holy Dying*, distinguishes carefully between human and divine healers: "You must give God thanks, and to the physician the honour of a blessed instrument" (127). Taylor further counsels his readers that they "use [physicians] temperately, without violent confidences" and cautions "that we be not too confident of the physician, or drain our hopes of recovery from the fountain through so imperfect channels" (127). Indeed, the danger of over-reliance on physicians is a constant theme in literature in nearly every era from Chaucer up to the twentieth century. So Lord John Hervey, in an eighteenth-century pathography that has not a trace of religious sentiment, cautions against placing one's trust in a physician, citing his eldest sister, who "had unfortunately (and the only flaw I knew in her understanding) faith in a physician . . . which ended, as the faith of a physician's votary generally does, in the ruin of herself and the discredit of her idol" (967). The parody of religious language in this enlightenment text is instructive. Even in a narrative devoid of religious sentiment, it is felt necessary to warn against inappropriate faith in a physician.

13. An important element in the success of Donne's blending of the religious and the medical is the fact that these two different disciplines were not so far apart in the seventeenth century. For example, it is difficult to determine whether some extant seventeenth-century tracts on illness are written by physicians or by clergymen: their shared vocabulary and the similarity in their conclusions makes them often indistinguishable (Slack, 255).

14. See Elizabeth Cox's *Thanksgiving*, discussed in chapter 5, a pathography about a husband with AIDS in which the authorial stance seems more inflected.

15. In fact, the serpent is mentioned in the *Devotions* in regard to its association with sin: "We are become devils to ourselves, and we have not only a serpent in our bosom, but we ourselves are to ourselves that serpent"; also, "sin . . . retains still so much of the author of it that it is a serpent, insensibly insinuating itself into my soul" (66, 69).

16. Though the pattern of Donne's conversion was remarkably similar to Augustine's —both changing from libertine to theologian—Donne produced no *Confessions:* it was left to Walton to recount, in what is as much hagiography as biography, Donne's extraordinary transformation. The *Devotions,* then, could be seen as a substitute for the spiritual autobiography Donne did not write, so that his sickness and recovery repeat in microcosm the larger pattern of his whole life.

Chapter 3: *Myths of Battle and Journey*

1. The stories of Greek mythology are rife with heroic journeys and battles with monsters: one thinks of Theseus making his way into the Cretan labyrinth to kill the minotaur, Orpheus in his journey into Hades to redeem Eurydice, or the wanderings of Heracles and his conquest of many monstrous adversaries. In the mythologies of the Celtic and Germanic peoples one also finds journeys into an "otherworld" where the hero triumphs over giants and witches, as in the exploits of the Welsh Culhwch or the Anglo-Saxon Beowulf.

2. Of course the *Iliad* is an exception, since it primarily concerns the battle between human combatants—the Achaians, and the Trojans and their allies. Homer here goes beyond the restrictions of the mythic paradigm in that the adversary is not perceived as monstrous or evil: indeed, Homer in some sense inverts the paradigm by creating a hero (Achilleus) who at times appears less than human, and an adversary (Hektor) who is the most fully human of all the characters in the poem. Too often, though, throughout the history of the West, a human enemy is (or has been) configured as subhuman in some way: our characterization in the twentieth century of the enemy as "Hun" or "Jap" is in this not so different from twelfth-century Christian notions of the Turk or the Infidel.

3. The briefest allusion to a non-Western philosophical model—the Chinese notion of Yin and Yang, for example—will by contrast highlight the Western tendency toward dualism. As the Chinese symbol for Yin-Yang demonstrates, such entities as light and dark, life and death (or sickness and health) are understood as complementary, not opposite attributes. Each, moreover, has a nucleus at its center of the opposite quality, suggesting that everything must contain within it the germ of its antithesis. Key here is the idea of complementary, not antagonistic principles, as in the West. Chinese medicine is based on just such a philosophical notion of complementarity: health is the consequence of a balance between the forces of Yin and Yang in the body; disease is an imbalance of these forces.

4. Susan Sontag, in her book on AIDS (1989), called popular attention to the use of military metaphor in descriptions of AIDS and its treatment.

5. The attempt to eradicate a disease is not dissimilar to the Calvinist endeavor to eradicate sin from one's life. Chemotherapy destroys the enemy cancer cells, but it attacks the host cells as well; "mortification," Calvin's remedy for sin, is effective as a spiritual therapy in that it destroys "our corrupt nature," but it also brings with it pain, suffering, and guilt (*Institutes*, 3.3.3.20, 672).

6. See the discussion in Chapter 2 on Terry Tempest Williams's *Refuge*, a pathography that questions the helpfulness of the military myth and suggests an alternative.

7. Howard Brody, in *Stories of Sickness* (137–42), offers a brief but interesting discussion of *Heartsounds* as an example of maladaptive ways of being sick.

8. The pathographies I discuss here are concerned exclusively with patients who contract AIDS through homosexual practices. Though this is a narrow sample of the actual population of AIDS patients, especially as the disease has evolved in recent years, it is representative of the genre at this time—exceptions being Fran Peavey's *A Shallow Pool of Time*, Elizabeth Glaser's *In the Absence of Angels*, Niro Asistent's *Why I Survive AIDS*, and several collections of pathographies, such as Andrea Rudd and Darien Taylor's *Positive Women*, Steven Petrow's *Dancing against the Darkness*, and Ines Rider and Patricia Ruppelt's *AIDS: The Women*. For a recent (and annotated) bibliography of AIDS pathographies, see Timothy F. Murphy and Suzanne Poirier, eds., *Writing AIDS: Gay Literature, Language, and Analysis*.

9. In contrast to most other pathographies, many of the books written about athletes, especially if they are professional athletes, are coauthored or the work of a professional writer. This to some extent may account for the tendency of these portraits to approximate eulogies.

10. Real life copies this goal of the heroic paradigm (at least in regard to motivating factors) in phenomena as diverse as Ponce de Leon's search for the Fountain of Youth, the alchemist's search for the philosopher's stone, or perhaps the search in medical science for the magic elixir, the magic talisman—the cure for cancer, or AIDS, or death.

11. What is striking about Sacks's pathography is not only that he likens his slow recovery to Dante's journey through Hell, Purgatory, and Heaven but that the original circumstances of Sacks's journey are so similar to the metaphorical frame in the *Divine Comedy*. The *Inferno* begins with Dante trying to climb a mountain, confronting three beasts who force him back down, falling into despair, and then meeting Virgil, who helps him reach his goal. Sacks's injury occurs when he is climbing a mountain, comes upon a bull, turns and runs away from it and then falls, tearing the quadriceps in his thigh. The difference between the two pilgrimages is the absence, for Sacks, of any figure such as Virgil to act as companion and guide in the journey back to health.

12. Anatole Broyard explicitly characterizes his "ideal doctor" as resembling Oliver Sacks, whom he knows through his writings (42–43).

13. A darker interpretation, suggested by one of my readers, is that patients often have myths imposed on them. This reader argues that it is in the institution's interest for patients to accept and acquiesce in the various "rites of passage" required, and in this way, myths can be seen as instruments of oppression rather than free and personal choices. It is my sense that the kind of hospital procedures I have discussed do have the character of ritual and do promote passivity and compliance, but they are fragmentary rituals that do not point toward any particular metaphoric construct: hospitals impose procedures, not myths. It is in the metaphoric interpretation of such rituals that a patient like Sacks can exercise creativity.

Chapter 4: *Constructing Death: Myths about Dying*

1. It is possible that the wide-scale appropriation of Elizabeth Kübler-Ross's articulated stages in the dying process functions as another way of denying death for some people, in that one's attention is deflected away from a focus on dying, itself, and onto an interpretive schema.

2. The death of Cato, who committed suicide rather than submit to the tyranny of Caesar, is also a famous and long-standing paradigm for the noble death. The poet Lucan wrote about Cato as a model of virtue, and before him, Cicero, in the *Tusculans,* linked the suicides of Cato and of Socrates. According to Plutarch, Socrates' death was actually used by Cato as the model for his own (Rist, 244).

3. The tendency to perceive dying and grieving as processes that occur in sequential and discrete stages is of course one result of the popularity of Kübler-Ross's influential *On Death and Dying*. It seems ironic that Meryman should indicate that "out of a sense of duty" he looked through a copy of *On Death and Dying* but found it irrelevant to his wife's situation (76).

4. During this period the author keeps a log of Carl's seizure activity and charts his cycles of improvement and deterioration. The ostensible purpose is to find patterns that might indicate whether certain symptoms are the result of the spreading tumor or side-effects of medication, but the deeper purpose seems to be that this act of recording helps her maintain some measure of detachment. In addition to her charts of symptoms and seizure activity, she cleans her home with an angry ferocity in an attempt to "banish [death] by meticulous neatness." "Order and precision" she observes, are "the signs of the cross that weaken [death's] power" (189). This need for "order and precision" she recognizes as an instinctive response to the unpredictable seizures—the random, disorderly movements of the cancer.

5. The continuing relevance of the book is borne out by the fact that it was reprinted in 1974, in paperback, with a fine introduction on euthanasia by Joseph Fletcher.

6. In the 1990s, with the recent publication of Derek Humphrey's *Final Exit* and the change in gender stereotypes effected by the feminist movement, the death by suicide of a terminal cancer patient is neither unusual nor particularly associated with the idea of manhood (see Betty Rollin's pathography, *Last Wish*, describing her mother's decision to end her life by an overdose of Nembutol rather than die slowly and painfully from cancer). It is of interest that the organizing myth in Rollin's pathography is closer to "easy death"—the myth often accompanying a pathographical description of a parent's death—than to "heroic" or "manly" death.

7. Beaty, 6, 25–31, discussing *The Boke of crafte of dyinge*.

8. In our century, when child mortality rates tend to be comparatively low, the death of a child can evoke more troubled questioning. In Camus's *The Plague*, the death of a child is described in polar contrast to Dickens's deathbed scenes: sheer physical torture, it is a justification for Rieux's metaphysical rebellion and the cause of Paneloux's religious despair.

9. Though this pathography was originally published in 1965 (the original, French version in 1964), the habit of not telling an elderly person that he or she is dying is still commonplace. Of course, in an age when death itself can be forestalled almost indefinitely, the very meaning of "dying" is called into question.

10. For a very different response to a similar situation, see de Beauvoir, 19–20.

Chapter 5: *Healthy-Mindedness: Myth as Medicine*

1. The term *holistic medicine* is often used as a synonym for alternative medicine and thus deserves further commentary. An attempt to synthesize mind and body, holistic medicine is actually more an approach to healing than a methodology. The term was coined in 1926 by Jan Smuts, a South African philosopher and politician who attempted to refute the reductionistic tendency of Darwinian evolution in an emphasis on the whole rather than its parts (Kopelman, 221). "Holism" for a long time designated an approach that considered all aspects of an individual's life—nutrition, life-style, environmental and social issues, emotional and spiritual well-being—to be relevant to his or her sickness, in contrast to biomedicine's tendency to focus exclusively on the malfunctioning body part or system. Jack LaPatra in 1978 remarked that holism is an approach emphasizing "the deep interdependence of body, mind, emotion, and spirit" (10). According to Kenneth Pelletier, holistic medicine "requires a consideration of all contributing factors: psychological,

psychosocial, environmental, and spiritual" (13). So described, a holistic approach can be compatible with the aims and methods of contemporary orthodox medicine—in fact, George Engel's "biopsychosocial model" suggests ways in which such an approach can be integrated into medicine.

More recently, the terms *holism* and *holistic healer* have been claimed by various practitioners of alternative medicine. And as such, the holistic approach has come to be associated with a particular philosophy of life. As David Teegarden writes in *The New Holistic Health Handbook,* "Holistic health is not merely the absence of disease. It is a state of well-being and vitality that brings about an optimal level of physical, mental, and spiritual functioning. In this state, you experience a sense of joy, wonder, and love toward your self and the world" (14). Similarly, Richard Miles observes that holistic health "focuses on the development of the joyful expression of good health, not on the achievement of normalcy or balance" (12). Not infrequently, holism connotes a responsibility not only to improve and maintain one's own health but also to work toward the well-being of all life forms. A holistic approach, then, suggests not just the interdependence of bodily, mental, emotional, and spiritual systems in the individual but a more global interdependence in an ecological and social awareness of the world in which we live and a strong sense of responsibility in working toward improving its health.

It is my belief that the medical profession should not allocate holism in health care to their rivals in alternative medicine. To do so is to encourage the belief that caring doctors—physicians who attend to the social, psychological, and spiritual dimensions of illness—cannot be found within orthodox medicine. This belief is the assumption underlying one pathographer's observation that a better alternative to today's orthodox medical model is "the holistic health model," in which the physician is "a skilled practitioner who must attend to caring as well as curing—to treating the whole person and focusing upon preventive medicine" (Simpson, 108–9). Though this author's remarks are meant simply as an endorsement of holistic medicine, they also serve as a serious indictment of contemporary biomedicine.

2. Alternative medicine can be seen not only as reactive, for those who use it, but also as revolutionary. Legally and economically biomedicine now exerts official control over health care in the United States: some forms of alternative medicine are illegal, there is no licensing procedure for most kinds of alternative practitioners, and funds for research in alternative medical treatments are virtually unavailable. In some sense, then, alternative medicine appears to be acting like an underground, grassroots movement—a force subverting the authority and hegemony of traditional medicine. The response of orthodox medicine has been varied: entrenchment in some quarters, especially in cancer therapy, where American citizens must cross the border into Mexico

if they choose to try certain alternative treatments, and compromise in others, such as the recent legitimization of an emphasis on diet, exercise, and stress reduction in treating heart disease.

3. My focus here is on the attitudes and beliefs that patients attach to illness and treatment. Some forms of alternative medicine are themselves constructs of healthy-mindedness: the various forms of visualization therapy, for example. But others, such as "straight" chiropractic, are not. Necessarily, my sample of contemporary alternative therapies is limited to those mentioned in the pathographies I have read.

4. The "sick soul" is characterized by the conviction that evil is an essential if deplorable aspect of one's self and world; the sense that nature is flawed and fallen and must be transcended; the recognition of guilt, sadness, and even despair as appropriate and potentially enabling emotions for a fallen self and world; and an equally relentless pessimism. My discussion of healthy-mindedness does not turn on the antithetical relationship of the "sick soul" and "healthy-mindedness." James was writing about religious experience, where the contrast seems genuinely illuminating. But to reduce medical experience to these two categories would most likely result in oversimplification and distortion.

5. David Hufford, in his OTA Contract Report for Selected Unorthodox Cancer Practitioners (Office of Technology Assessment, U.S. Congress, May 1988), finds that there has been a consistent rise in New Age thought, which in many ways is quite close to healthy-mindedness, at least since the time of Emerson and Thoreau in the early 1800s.

6. Some examples are Alice Elaine Cler's *Cancer, God, and I, and a Natural Cure,* Eydie Mae Hunsberger's *How I Conquered Cancer Naturally,* and Beata Bishop's *A Triumph over Cancer.* Each concerns a woman diagnosed with cancer and each advocates a naturopathic therapy. These pathographies all share the conviction that illness is the result of an accumulation of toxins in the body—toxins acquired principally from chemical additives in food, but also from exposure to radiation and from breathing air contaminated with pollutants. In short, civilized life is felt to be toxic, and toxins are believed to cause disease. Recovery entails purifying the body of the poisons of civilization, and the principle way of doing so is by eating foods that are organic, unprocessed, raw, or fresh.

   The most common pattern in these pathographies is that the patient develops cancer; finds orthodox medical treatment unsatisfactory or rejects it outright; discovers, usually through the media, some form of naturopathic cure; and in the end, experiences a dramatic reversal of symptoms. At first, these pathographies seem similar to those I have been calling "healthy-minded," in that they describe the author's (usually successful) experimentation with some form of alternative medicine. But they differ from their healthy-minded counterparts in their emphasis first, on dietary issues, and only secondarily, on the psychological aspects of illness and recovery; they also differ in the distrust (sometimes hostility) that their authors direct toward the medical establishment. In pathographies governed by the healthy-minded mythos, most patients combine alternative therapies with orthodox medicine. But a purification diet is almost never undertaken in concert with orthodox medicine; most often the naturopathic cure substitutes for conventional medical therapy.

Of course there is some overlap between healthy-minded pathographies and those advocating dietary treatments: Norman Cousins's *Anatomy of an Illness* begins with a recognition of the deleterious effect of environmental pollutants on the immune system, and Laura Chester in *Lupus Novice* describes her extensive experimentation with naturopathic remedies: both are pathographies I discuss as examples of healthy-mindedness. Conversely, Beata Bishop in her pathography describes her successful recovery from melanoma by rigorously following Gerson therapy (a strict vegetarian diet with large amounts of raw fruit juice, periodic injections of crude liver, and frequent coffee enemas), which she supplements with Simonton image-therapy.

Readers interested in dietary pathographies will want to look at Anthony Sattilaro's *Recalled by Life*. The author is a physician with metastatic prostate cancer who supplements conventional medical treatments with a strict macrobiotic diet. Sattilaro's attempt throughout the book to balance his experiential knowledge as a patient and the scientific medical model which he espouses as a physician is striking. In *Recovery from Cancer to Health through Macrobiotics,* Elaine Nussbaum cites Sattilaro's pathography as the source of her knowledge about the link between macrobiotics and cancer and as providing her with the impetus to experiment with a macrobiotic diet: "The doctor [Sattilaro] had been riddled with cancer, and now he was well. 'If he could do it,' I said to myself, 'Why can't I?'" (130). Nussbaum is diagnosed as having endometrial cancer with metastases to both lungs and the spine, which is treated with surgery, chemotherapy, and radiation. After six months of a macrobiotic diet supplemented with shiatsu treatments, she "had changed drastically—from a sick, depressed, pill-popping invalid to a happy, optimistic, pain-free, and a very grateful woman" (177). Unlike Sattilaro and Nussbaum, Dirk Benedict, in *Confessions of a Kamikaze Cowboy,* repeatedly expresses open hostility toward "that contemporary institutionalized witchcraft known as the medical establishment" (xxi) while telling his story of curing what he assumes to be prostate cancer by means of a strict macrobiotic diet.

A good overview of popular dietary therapies—one based on the experience of the patients who use and have benefited from them—can be found in Judith Glassman's *The Cancer Survivors.*

7. Louise Hay (*You Can Heal Your Life*) is for AIDS patients what the Simontons and Bernie Siegel are for cancer patients. A healthy-minded pathography that illustrates (and discusses) Hay's approach at length is Louie Nassaney's *I Am Not a Victim.*

8. The terms *optimists* and *realists* come from *Head First.*

9. In *Head First*, Cousins is much more emphatic than in his earlier book in asserting a causal relationship between attitude and recovery. Thus he writes: "Nothing was more striking than the fact that far more optimists were able to conquer their illness than were the 'realists'" (14).

10. More recent books by the Simontons on the psychological causes and treatment of cancer are Stephanie Matthews Simonton's *The Healing Family* (1984), which focuses on the role the family can play in helping a loved one deal with and recover from cancer, and O. Carl Simonton's *The Healing Journey* (1992), coauthored with a patient, Reid Henson—a book that is itself a pathography illustrating the Simonton approach to cancer treatment.

11. In the medical system of any culture, it is usually assumed that a particular therapy need not necessarily be fully understood by the patient for it to be effective. But one must not go on to assume that any such therapy is efficacious simply in itself. Belief and cultural consensus are of paramount importance: patients who submit to the orthodox medical therapies of their culture do so because they believe these therapies will be effective and because of the force of cultural habit. Such cultural compulsion is a highly significant factor in cure, as we know from research confirming the placebo effect.

12. Extensive doctor-shopping is not restricted to those who experiment with alternative medicine; it is also common to pathographies in which patients research and then "shop" for state-of-the-art cancer research protocols. Barbara Creaturo, who uses the National Cancer Center's "hotline" to identify promising experimental treatments, observes: "In the absence of any consensus about how my malignancy [ovarian cancer] might be best treated, I had to become a student of my disease, checking one therapy against another, shopping for my cure, and, ultimately, the arbiter of my own treatment" (250).

13. As the interviews in Michael Callen's *Surviving AIDS* demonstrate, many people with AIDS complement orthodox treatment with alternative therapies. To some extent, this pattern reflects the mistrust with which the homosexual community views the efforts of biomedicine and the federal government to find a valid treatment for AIDS. The approval of AZT, for example, is perceived by Callen as "a scandal of the magnitude of thalidomide" (216). According to Callen, and to many of the individuals with AIDS whom he interviews, AZT is neither safe nor effective.

14. The Simontons advocate the use of meditation and visualizations as supplementary to traditional medical therapies, not as a substitution for it. In this

pathography, Virginia Hine observes that "Carl [Simonton] supported Aldie's decision to delay physical therapy" (40).

15. This early picture of the way Radner oscillates between orthodox and alternative medicine during the initial stages of her illness in fact becomes a pattern, repeated again and again as the narrative and the illness progress. The notion of a patient, like "Everyman" in a medieval morality play, poised between opposing systems of health care treatment (orthodox and alternative) may seem anomalous to some readers, but a survey of pathographical narratives indicates that this may be the way many people today deal with their medical needs. Max Lerner, for example, diagnosed as having large cell lymphoma in an advanced state, devotes an entire chapter, called "The Torment of Choice," to the process whereby he chooses between "the bruising effect of medical technology" that goes along with orthodox cancer treatments and "the still dubious alternative treatments" (42).

Afterword

1. Autobiographical documents of illness as experienced by the poor are beginning to appear: see chapter 1, note 2.

2. Examples of this kind of writing are some of John Stone's poems and essays, Perri Klass's *Other Women's Children,* and David Hilfiker's *Healing the Wounds.*

✟

Achterberg, Jeanne, and G. Frank Lawlis. *Imagery of Cancer.* Champaign, Ill.: Institute for Personality and Ability Testing, 1978.

Aladjem, Henrietta. *The Sun Is My Enemy: One Woman's Victory over a Mysterious and Dreaded Disease.* Englewood Cliffs, N.J.: Prentice-Hall, 1972; reissued as *In Search of the Sun: A Woman's Courageous Victory over Lupus,* with Peter H. Schur, rev. ed. 1988, Macmillan.

Ariès, Philippe. *Western Attitudes toward Death.* Translated by P. M. Ranum. Baltimore, Md.: Johns Hopkins University Press, 1974.

Aristotle. *Nicomachean Ethics: The Basic Works of Aristotle.* Edited by R. McKeon. New York: Random House, 1941.

Asistent, Niro Markoff, with Paul Duffy. *Why I Survive AIDS.* New York: Fireside; Simon & Schuster, 1991.

Atwood, Dave. *Tomorrow Is a Better Day.* New York: Vantage, 1986.

Augustine. *Confessions.* 2 vols. Translated by W. Watts, revised by W. H. D. Rouse. Loeb Classical Library. Cambridge, Mass.: Harvard University Press; London, England: Heinemann, 1977.

Baier, Sue, and Mary Zimmeth. *Bed Number Ten.* New York: Holt, Rinehart and Winston, 1986.

Bailey, Thomas. *Voices of America.* New York: Free Press, 1976.

Banks, Sam A. "Once Upon a Time: Interpretation in Literature and Medicine." *Literature and Medicine* 1 (1982): 23–27.

Baron, Richard. "Bridging Clinical Distance: An Empathic Rediscovery of the Known." *Journal of Medicine and Philosophy* 6, no. 1 (Fall 1981): 5–23.

Beaty, Nancy Lee. *The Craft of Dying: A Study in the Literary Tradition of the Ars Moriendi in England.* New Haven, Conn.: Yale University Press, 1970.

Beauvoir, Simone de. *A Very Easy Death.* Translated by Patrick O'Brien. New York: Pantheon, 1965; 1985.

Benedict, Dirk. *Confessions of a Kamikaze Cowboy.* North Hollywood, Calif.: Newcastle Publishing Co. Inc., 1987.

Berté, Raymond A. *To Speak Again: Victory over Cancer.* Agawam, Mass.: Phillips Publishing Company, 1987.

Bishop, Beata. *My Triumph over Cancer: The Therapy of the Future.* New Canaan, Conn.: Keats Publishing Company, 1986 (published by Severn House Publishers, 1985, as *A Time to Heal*).

Blair, Barbara, and Susan E. Cayliff. *Wings of Gauze: Women of Color and the Experience of Health and Illness.* Detroit, Mich.: Wayne State University Press, 1993.

Blakely, Mary Kay. *Wake Me When It's Over: A Journey to the Edge and Back.* New York: Times Books, 1989.

Bliss, Shepherd, ed. *The New Holistic Health Handbook.* Lexington, Ky.: Stephen Green Press, 1985.

Bloch, Richard and Annette. *Cancer . . . There's Hope.* Kansas City, Mo.: The Cancer Connection Inc., 1981.

Blumberg, Rena. *Headstrong: A Story of Conquests and Celebrations . . . Living through Chemotherapy.* New York: Crown Publishing, Inc., 1982.

Bodkin, Maud. *Archetypal Patterns in Poetry: Psychological Studies in Imagination.* New York: Vintage, 1958.

Braudy, Leo. "Daniel Defoe and the Anxieties of Autobiography." *Genre* 6, no. 1 (March 1973): 76–97.

Brée, Germaine, "Michel Leiris: Mazemaker." In *Autobiography,* edited by Olney (which see), 194–206.

Brody, Howard. *Stories of Sickness.* New Haven, Conn.: Yale University Press, 1987.

Brown, H. C. *Walking toward Your Fear.* Nashville, Tenn.: Broadman, 1972.

Broyard, Anatole. *Intoxicated by My Illness and Other Writings on Life and Death,* edited by Alexandra Broyard. New York: Clarkson Potter, 1992. [Contains essays reprinted from the *New York Times Magazine* and the *New York Times Book Review.*]

Bruss, Elizabeth. *Autobiographical Acts: The Changing Situation of a Literary Genre.* Baltimore, Md.: Johns Hopkins University Press, 1976.

Buchanan, William. *A Shining Season.* New York: Bantam, 1978.

Bultmann, Rudolf. "New Testament and Mythology." In *New Testament and Mythology and Other Basic Writings,* translated and edited by Schubert M. Ogden. Philadelphia, Pa.: Fortress Press, 1984.

Bunyan, John. *Grace Abounding to the Chief of Sinners.* Edited by Roger Sharrock. Oxford, England: Clarendon Press, 1966.

Butler, Sandra, and Barbara Rosenblum. *Cancer in Two Voices.* San Francisco, Calif.: Spinsters Book Co., 1991.

Callen, Michael. *Surviving AIDS.* New York: Harper Perennial, 1990.

Calvin, John. *Institutes of the Christian Religion.* 2 vols. Translated by John Allen. Philadelphia, Pa.: Westminster Press, 1813.

Campbell, Joseph. *The Hero with a Thousand Faces.* New York: Meridian Books, 1956.

Carter, Albert Howard III. "Metaphors in the Physician-Patient Relationship." *Soundings* 72, no. 1 (Spring 1989): 153–63.

Cassell, Eric J. *The Nature of Suffering and the Goals of Medicine.* New York: Oxford University Press, 1991.

Cassirer, Ernst. *The Philosophy of Symbolic Forms.* Vol. 2, *Mythical Thought.* Translated by Ralph Manheim. New Haven, Conn.: Yale University Press, 1955.

Castelli, Jim. *I'm Too Young to Have a Heart Attack.* Rochlen, Calif.: Prime Publishing Company, 1990.

Charon, Rita. "To Render the Lives of Patients." *Literature and Medicine* 5 (1986): 58–74.

———. "Doctor-Patient/Reader-Writer: Learning to Find the Text." *Soundings* 72, no. 1 (Spring 1989): 137–52.

Chester, Laura. *Lupus Novice: Toward Self-Healing.* Barrytown, N.Y.: Station Hill Press, 1987.

Churchill, Larry R. "The Human Experience of Dying: The Moral Primacy of Stories over Stages." *Soundings* 42, no. 1 (Spring 1979): 24–37.

Clark, Eleanor. *Eyes, Etc.: A Memoir.* New York: Pantheon, 1977.

Cler, Alice Elaine, and Barbara Cler Pendleton. *Cancer, God, and I, and a Natural Cure.* New York: Vantage, 1987.

Conley, Herbert N. *Living and Dying Gracefully.* New York: Paulist Press, 1979.

Cook, Stephanie. *Second Life.* New York: Simon and Schuster, 1981.

Cousins, Norman. "Anatomy of an Illness (as Perceived by the Patient)." *New England Journal of Medicine* 295 (23 December, 1976): 1458–63.

———. *Anatomy of an Illness as Perceived by the Patient.* New York: Norton, 1979.

Cousins, Norman. *The Healing Heart: Antidotes to Panic and Helplessness.* New York: Norton, 1983.

———. *Head First: The Biology of Hope.* New York: E. P. Dutton, 1989.

Cowie, Bill. "The Cardiac Patient's Perception of His Heart Attack." *Social Science and Medicine* 10, no. 2 (February 1976): 87–96.

Cox, Elizabeth. *Thanksgiving: An AIDS Journal.* New York: Harper and Row, 1990.

Cox, James M. *Recovering Literature's Lost Ground: Essays in American Autobiography.* Baton Rouge, La., and London, England: Louisiana State University Press, 1989.

Craig, Jean. *Between Hello & Goodbye: A Life-Affirming Story of Courage in the Face of Tragedy.* Los Angeles, Calif.: Jeremy P. Tarcher, Inc., 1991.

Creaturo, Barbara. *Courage: The Testimony of a Cancer Patient.* New York: Pantheon, 1991.

Dardel, Eric. "The Mythic." *Diogenes* 7 (Summer 1954): 33–51.

Davison, Jaquie. *Cancer Winner: How I Purged Myself of Melanoma.* Pierce City, Mo.: Pacific Press, 1977.

Donne, John. *Devotions upon Emergent Occasions.* Ann Arbor: University of Michigan Press, 1959.

Dravecky, Dave and Jan, with Ken Gire. *When You Can't Come Back.* Grand Rapids, Mich.: Zondervan Publishing House; San Francisco, Calif.: HarperSanFrancisco, 1992.

Dravecky, Dave, and Tim Stafford. *Comeback.* Grand Rapids, Mich.: Zondervan Publishing House; San Francisco, Calif.: Harper and Row, 1990.

Dreuilhe, Emmanuel. *Mortal Embrace: Living with AIDS.* Translated by Linda Coverdale. New York: Hill and Wang; Farrar, Straus and Giroux, 1988.

Duclow, David. "Dying on Broadway: Contemporary Drama on Mortality." *Soundings* 64, no. 2 (Summer 1981): 195–216.

Eakin, Paul John. *Fictions in Autobiography: Studies in the Art of Self-Invention.* Princeton, N.J.: Princeton University Press, 1985.

Elbaz, Robert. *The Changing Nature of the Self: A Critical Study of the Autobiographic Discourse.* Iowa City: University of Iowa Press, 1987.

Eliade, Mircea. *Rites and Symbols of Initiation: The Mysteries of Birth and Rebirth.* Translated by Willard R. Trask. New York: Harper and Row, 1958.

Engel, George L. "The Need for a New Medical Model: A Challenge for Bio-medicine." *Science* 196 (1977): 129–36

———. "The Clinical Application of the Biopsychosocial Model." *American Journal of Psychiatry* 137 (1980): 535–44.

Epstein, Alice Hopper. *Mind, Fantasy and Healing: One Woman's Journey from Conflict and Illness to Wholeness and Health.* New York: Delacorte; Bantam, 1989.

Farnsworth, Ken. *The Ultimate Healing.* Wilton, Conn.: Morehouse Publishing Co., 1989.

Fiore, Neil A. *The Road Back to Health: Coping with the Emotional Side of Cancer.* Toronto, Canada: Bantam, 1984.

Frank, Arthur W. *At the Will of the Body: Reflections on Illness.* Boston, Mass.: Houghton Mifflin Co., 1991.

Freud, Sigmund. *Leonardo da Vinci and a Memory of His Childhood.* Translated by Alan Tyson. New York: W. W. Norton and Company, 1964

Friedman, Meyer, and Ray H. Rosenman. *Type A Behavior and Your Heart.* New York: Alfred Knopf, 1974.

Gennep, Arnold van. *The Rites of Passage.* Translated by Monika B. Vizedom and Gabrielle L. Caffee. Chicago, Ill.: University of Chicago Press, 1960.

Girouard, Mark. *The Return to Camelot: Chivalry and the English Gentleman.* New Haven, Conn.: Yale University Press, 1981.

Glaser, Elizabeth, and Laura Palmer. *In the Absence of Angels: A Hollywood Family's Courageous Story.* New York: G. P. Putnam, 1991.

Glassman, Judith. *The Cancer Survivors and How They Did It.* New York: The Dial Press/Doubleday & Co., 1983.

Goshen-Gottstein, Esther. *Recalled to Life: The Story of a Coma.* New Haven, Conn.: Yale University Press, 1990.

Graham, Jory. *In the Company of Others.* New York: Harcourt Brace Jovanovich, 1982.

Greer, Virginia. *The Glory Woods: A Hymn of Healing.* Chappaqua, N.Y.: Christian Herald House, 1976.

Hargrove, Anne C. *Getting Better: Conversations with Myself and Other Friends While Healing from Breast Cancer.* Minneapolis, Minn.: CompCare Publishers, 1988.

Hawkins, Anne Hunsaker. "Two Pathographies: A Study in Illness and Literature." *Journal of Medicine and Philosophy* 9, no. 3 (August 1984): 231–52.

———. *Archetypes of Conversion: The Spiritual Autobiographies of Augustine, Bunyan, and Merton.* Lewisburg, Pa.: Bucknell University Press, 1985.

———. "A Change of Heart: The Paradigm of Regeneration in Medical and Religious Narrative." *Perspectives in Biology and Medicine* 33, no. 4 (Summer 1990): 547–59.

———. "Constructing Death: Three Pathographies about Dying." *Omega* 22, no. 4 (1991): 301–17.

———. "Charting Dante: The Inferno and Medical Education." *Literature and Medicine* 11, no. 2 (Fall 1992): 200–215.

———. "Restoring the Patient's Voice: The Case of Gilda Radner," *Yale Journal of Biology and Medicine* 65, no. 4 (1992): in press.

Hay, Louise L. *You Can Heal Your Life.* Santa Monica, Calif.: Hay House, 1984.

Helman, Ethel. *An Autumn Life: How a Surgeon Faced His Fatal Illness.* London, England: Faber and Faber, 1986.

Hervey, Lord John. "An Account of My Own Constitution and Illness, with Some Rules for the Preservation of Health; for the Use of My Children" (1731). In *Some Materials towards Memoirs of the Reign of King George II,* vol. 3, edited by Romney Sedgwick. Appendix 2, 961–87. New York: AMS Press; London, England: King's, 1931.

Hickey, Des, with Gus Smith. *Miracle.* London: Hodder and Stoughton, 1978.

Hilfiker, David. *Healing the Wounds: A Physician Looks at His Work.* New York: Pantheon, 1985.

Hine, Virginia. *Last Letter to the Pebble People: "Aldie Soars."* Santa Cruz, Calif.: Unity Press, 1977.

Hingle, Patricia. *A Coming of Roses.* Prairieville, La.: Home Plates of Ascension, 1988.

Homer. *The Iliad.* Translated by Richard Lattimore. Chicago, Ill.: University of Chicago Press, 1951.

Hostetler, Helen M. *A Time to Love.* Scottdale, Pa.: Herald Press, 1989.

Howe, Herbert M. *Do Not Go Gentle.* New York: Norton, 1981.

Hufford, David. "Contemporary Folk Medicine." In *Other Healers: Unorthodox Medicine in America,* edited by Norman Gevitz. Baltimore, Md., and London, England: Johns Hopkins University Press, 1988.

Humphrey, Derek. *Final Exit.* Eugene, Oreg.: Hemlock Society, 1992.

Humphrey, Derek, with Ann Wickett. *Jean's Way.* New York: Quartet Books, 1978. Reprint. New York: Harper & Row/Perennial, 1986.

Hunsberger, Eydie Mae, with Chris Loeffler. *How I Conquered Cancer Naturally.* Irving, Calif.: Harvest House Publishers, 1975. Reprint. Garden City Park, N.Y.: Avery Publishing Group, Inc., 1992.

Hunter, Kathryn Montgomery. "A Science of Individuals: Medicine and Casuistry." *The Journal of Medicine and Philosophy* 14 (1989): 193–212.

————. *Doctors' Stories: The Narrative Structure of Medical Knowledge.* Princeton, N.J.: Princeton University Press, 1991.

Ireland, Jill. *Life Wish.* Boston, Mass.: Little, Brown and Company, 1987.

James, William. *The Varieties of Religious Experience.* New York: Mentor; New American Library, 1958.

Johnson, James L. *Coming Back: One Man's Journey to the Edge of Eternity and Spiritual Rediscovery.* N.p.: Springhouse, 1979.

Johnson, Lois Walfred. *Either Way I Win: A Guide for Growth in the Power of Prayer.* Minneapolis, Minn.: Augsburg Publishing House, 1979.

Jones, Anne Hudson. "Metaphors, Narratives, and Images of AIDS." *Medical Humanities Review* 4, no. 1 (January 1990): 7–16.

Jones, Terry L., and David F. Nixon. *Venom in My Veins: One Man's Battle against Lou Gehrig's Disease.* Kansas City, Mo.: Beacon Hill Press, 1985.

Kastenbaum, Robert and Beatrice. *The Encyclopedia of Death.* Phoenix, Ariz.: Oryx Press, 1989.

Kastenbaum, Robert, and Ruth Aisenberg. *The Psychology of Death.* New York: Springer Publication Company, 1972.

Kavinoky, Bernice. *Voyage and Return.* New York: Norton, 1966.

Keiser, Bea, with Janice Booker. *All Our Hearts Are Trump.* Durham, N. C.: Moore Publishing Company, 1976.

Klass, Perri. *Other Women's Children.* New York: Random House, 1990.

Kleinman, Arthur. *The Illness Narratives.* New York: Basic Books, 1988.

Kolakowski, Leszek. *The Presence of Myth.* Translated by Adam Czerniawski. Chicago, Ill., and London, England: University of Chicago Press, 1989.

Kopelman, Loretta, and John Moskop. "The Holistic Health Movement: A Survey and Critique." *The Journal of Medicine and Philosophy* 6 (1981): 209–35.

Kübler-Ross, Elisabeth. *On Death and Dying.* New York: Macmillan, 1969.

LaPatra, Jack. *Healing.* New York: McGraw-Hill, 1978.

Lear, Martha Weinman. *Heartsounds: The Story of a Love and Loss.* New York: Simon and Schuster, 1980.

Lee, Laurel. *Walking through the Fire: A Hospital Journal.* New York: Dutton, 1977.

————. *Signs of Spring.* New York: E. P. Dutton, 1980.

Lejeune, Philippe. *On Autobiography.* Translated by Katherine Lear and edited by Paul John Eakin. Minneapolis, Minn.: University of Minnesota Press, 1989.

Lerner, Gerda. *A Death of One's Own.* New York: Simon and Schuster, 1978.

Lerner, Max. *Wrestling with the Angel: A Memoir of My Triumph over Illness.* New York: W. W. Norton, 1990.

Levine, Louis S. *Heart Attack.* New York: Harper and Row, 1976.

Lifton, Robert Jay. *Death in Life: Survivors of Hiroshima.* New York: Random House, 1967.

————. *The Broken Connection.* New York: Simon and Schuster, 1979.

Lorde, Audre. *The Cancer Journals.* Argyle, N.Y.: Spinsters, Ink *[sic]*, 1980.

Lund, Doris. *Eric.* New York: Laurel-Leaf Library Book; Dell, 1974.

Lyons, John O. *The Invention of the Self: The Hinge of Consciousness in the Eighteenth Century.* Carbondale: Southern Illinois University Press, 1978.

McDowell, Mildred. *Open Heart.* New York: Paulist Press, 1978.

Macherey, Pierre. *A Theory of Literary Production.* Translated by Geoffrey Wall. London, England, and Boston, Mass.: Routledge and Kegan Paul, 1978.

Madruga, Lenor. *One Step at a Time: A Young Woman's Inspiring Struggle to Walk Again.* New York: Signet; McGraw-Hill, 1979.

Mandel, Barrett John. "Autobiography—Reflection Trained on Mystery." *Prairie Schooner* 46 (1972): 323–38.

————. "Full of Life Now." In *Autobiography,* edited by Olney (which see), 49–72.

Mandell, Arnold J. *Coming of Middle Age: A Journey.* New York: Summit, 1977.

Mandell, Harvey, and Howard Spiro. *When Doctors Get Sick.* New York and London: Plenum Medical Book Co., 1987.

Mattsson, Gunnar. *The Princess.* Translated by Joan Bulman. New York: Dutton, 1967.

Melton, George R. *Beyond AIDS: A Journey into Healing.* Beverly Hills, Calif.: Brotherhood Press, 1988.

Merton, Thomas. *The Seven Storey Mountain.* New York: Harcourt Brace and Company, 1948.

Meryman, Richard. *Hope: A Loss Survived.* Boston, Mass.: Little, Brown and Company, 1980.

Metzger, Deena. "Tree." In *The Woman Who Slept with Men & Tree.* Berkeley, Calif.: Wingbow Press, 1978; 1981.

Michael, Peter Paul. *Multiple Sclerosis: A Dragon with a Hundred Heads.* Port Washington, N.Y.: Ashley Books, 1981.

Miles, Richard B. "Humanistic Medicine and Holistic Health Care." In *The New Holistic Health Handbook,* edited by Bliss (which see), 8–13.

Mille, Agnes de. *Reprieve: A Memoir.* New York: Doubleday, 1981.

Mishler, Elliot G. *The Discourse of Medicine: Dialectics of Medical Interviews.* Norwood, N.J.: Ablex Publishing Corporation,1984.

Mitchell, Joyce Slayton. *Winning the Chemo Battle.* New York: W. W. Norton, 1988.

Monette, Paul. *Borrowed Time: An AIDS Memoir.* San Diego, Calif.: Harcourt Brace Jovanovich, 1988.

Morris, Jeannie. *Brian Piccolo: A Short Season.* New York: Dell, 1971.

Morris, John N. *Versions of the Self: Studies in English Autobiography from John Bunyan to John Stuart Mill.* New York: Basic Books, 1966.

Mullan, Fitzhugh. *Vital Signs: A Young Doctor's Struggle with Cancer.* New York: Farrar, Straus, Giroux, 1982.

Murphy, Robert. *The Body Silent.* New York: Henry Holt and Company, 1987.

Murphy, Timothy F., and Suzanne Poirier, eds. *Writing AIDS: Gay Literature, Language, and Analysis.* New York: Columbia University Press, 1993.

Nassaney, Louie, with Glenn Kolb. *I Am Not a Victim: One Man's Triumph over Fear and AIDS.* Santa Monica, Calif.: Hay House, Inc., 1990.

Nolan, William. *Surgeon under the Knife.* New York: Coward, McCann and Geoghegan, 1976.

Noll, Peter. *In the Face of Death.* Translated by Hans Noll. New York: Viking; Penguin, 1989.

Norris, Patricia, and Garrett Porter. *Why Me? Harnessing the Healing Power of the Human Spirit.* Walpole, N.H.: Stillpoint Publishing Company,1985.

Nussbaum, Elaine. *Recovery from Cancer to Health through Macrobiotics.* Tokyo and New York: Japan Publications Inc., 1986.

Oden, Clifford. *Thank God I Have Cancer!* New Rochelle, N.Y.: Arlington House, 1976.

Olney, Richard. *Metaphors of Self: The Meaning of Autobiography.* Princeton, N.J.: Princeton University Press. 1972.

————, ed. *Autobiography: Essays Theoretical and Critical.* Princeton, N.J.: Princeton University Press, 1980.

Olsen, Kristin Gottschalk. *The Encyclopedia of Alternative Health Care.* New York: Simon and Schuster; Pocket Books, 1989.

Owen, Bob. *Roger's Recovery from AIDS.* Malibu, Calif.: DAVAR, 1987.

Panger, Daniel. *The Dance of the Wild Mouse.* Glen Ellen, Calif.: Entwhistle Books, 1979.

Paoli, Pia. *Determined to Live.* Translated by Diana Athill. New York: Harcourt, 1968.

Pascal, Roy. *Design and Truth in Autobiography.* Cambridge, Mass.: Harvard University Press, 1960.

Payer, Lynn. *Medicine and Culture: Varieties of Treatments in the United States, England, West Germany, and France.* New York: Henry Holt and Company, 1988.

Peabody, Barbara. *The Screaming Room.* San Diego, Calif.: Oak Tree Publishing Company, 1986.

Pearson, Carol Lynn. *Good-Bye, I Love You.* New York: Random House, 1986.

Peavey, Fran. *A Shallow Pool of Time: An HIV+ Woman Grapples with the AIDS Epidemic.* Philadelphia, Pa.: New Society Publishers, 1990.

Pelgrin, Mark. *And a Time to Die.* Edited by Sheila Moon and Elizabeth B. Howes. Wheaton, Ill.: Theosophical Publishing House, 1962.

Pelletier, Kenneth R. *Holistic Medicine.* New York: Delacorte, 1979.

Pepper, Curtis Bill. *We the Victors.* New York: Doubleday, 1984.

Permut, Joanna Baumer. *Embracing the Wolf: A Lupus Victim and Her Family Learn to Live with Chronic Disease.* Atlanta, Ga.: Cherokee Publishing Company, 1989.

Perry, Shireen, and Gregg Lewis. *In Sickness and in Health: A Story of Love in the Shadow of AIDS*. Downers Grove, Ill.: Intervarsity Press, 1989.

Petrow, Steven. *Dancing against the Darkness: Journeys through America in the Age of AIDS*. Lexington, Mass.: D. C. Heath and Co., 1990.

Photopulos, Georgia and Bud. *Of Tears and Triumphs*. New York: Congdon & Weed, Inc., 1987.

Pike, Burton. "Time in Autobiography." *Comparative Literature* 28 (1976): 326–42.

Plato. *Laws*. Translated by B. Jowett. In *The Dialogues of Plato*, vol. 2. New York: Random House, 1892.

———. *Phaedo*. Translated by F. J. Church. Liberal Arts Press. Indianapolis, Ind.: Bobbs-Merrill, 1951.

———. *Euthyphro*. Translated by F. J. Church. Library of Liberal Arts. Indianapolis, Ind.: Bobbs-Merrill, 1956.

Pond, Jean. *Surviving*. New York: Ace Books, 1978.

Priest, Mary Woodward. *Diary of Courage: Coping with Life-Threatening Illness*. San Francisco, Calif.: Strawberry Hill Press, 1990.

Radner, Gilda. *It's Always Something*. New York: Avon Books, 1989.

Radziunas, Eileen. *Lupus: My Search for a Diagnosis*. Edited by Jackie Melvin. Claremont, Calif.: Hunter House, 1989.

Reinfeld, Nyles V. *Open Heart Surgery: A Second Chance*. Englewood Cliffs, N.J.: Prentice-Hall, 1983.

Renza, Louis. "The Veto of the Imagination: A Theory of Autobiography." In *Autobiography*, edited by Olney (which see), 268–95.

Rider, Ines, and Patricia Ruppelt, eds. *AIDS: The Women*. San Francisco, Calif.: Cleis, 1988.

Rist, J. M. *Stoic Philosophy*. Cambridge, England: Cambridge University Press, 1969.

Robinson, Eric. *One Dark Mile: A Widower's Story*. Amherst: University of Massachusetts Press, 1989.

Rodale, Ardath H. *Climbing toward the Light*. Emmaus, Pa.: Good Spirit Press, 1989.

Rollin, Betty. *First You Cry*. Philadelphia, Pa.: J. B. Lippincott, 1976.

Rollin, Betty. *Last Wish.* New York: Warner Books, 1985.

Rosenbaum, Edward E. *A Taste of My Own Medicine: When the Doctor Is the Patient.* New York: Random House, 1988.

Ross, Judith Wilson. "The Militarization of Disease: Do We Really Want a War on AIDS?" *Soundings* 72, no. 1 (Spring 1989): 39–58.

Rossi, Nancy. *From This Day Forward: A True Love Story.* New York: Times Books, 1983.

Roth, Philip. *Patrimony: A True Story.* New York: Simon and Schuster, 1991.

Rousseau, G. S. "Literature and Medicine: Toward a Simultaneity of Theory and Practice." *Literature and Medicine* 5 (1986): 152–81.

Rudd, Andrea, and Darien Taylor. *Positive Women: Views of Women Living with AIDS.* Toronto: Second Story Press, 1992.

Ryan, Cornelius. *A Bridge Too Far.* New York: Simon and Schuster, 1974.

Ryan, Cornelius, and Kathryn Morgan Ryan. *A Private Battle.* New York: Fawcett, 1979.

Sacks, Oliver. *Awakenings.* New York: Harper Perennial, 1990; New York: Dutton, 1983.

———. *A Leg to Stand On.* New York: Summit Books, 1984.

———. *The Man Who Mistook His Wife for a Hat.* New York: Summit Books, 1985.

Sarton, May. *After the Stroke: A Journal.* New York: Norton, 1988.

Sattilaro, Anthony, and Tom Monte. *Recalled by Life: The Story of My Recovery from Cancer.* Boston, Mass.: Houghton Mifflin, 1982.

Schreiber, Le Anne. *Midstream.* New York: Viking Penguin, 1990.

Schwerin, Doris. *Diary of a Pigeon Watcher.* New York: William Morrow and Company, 1976.

Secundy, Marian Gray, ed. *Trials, Tribulations, and Celebrations: African-American Perspectives on Health, Illness, Aging, and Loss.* Yarmouth, Me.: Intercultural Press, 1992.

Segal, Robert A. "In Defense of Mythology: The History of Modern Theories of Myth." *Annals of Scholarship* 1 (1980): 3–49.

Shapero, Lucy, and Anthony A. Goodman. *Never Say Die: A Doctor and Patient Talk about Breast Cancer.* New York: Appleton, 1980.

Shapiro, Kenneth A. *Dying and Living: One Man's Life with Cancer.* Austin: University of Texas Press, 1985.

Sharrock, Roger. *John Bunyan.* London, England: Hutchinson's University Library, 1954.

Shook, Robert L. *Survivors: Living with Cancer.* New York: Harper and Row, 1983.

Siegel, Bernie S. *The Healing Power of Love and Laughter* (sound recording). Edena, Minn.: Effective Learning Systems, 1983.

———. *Love, Medicine and Miracles.* New York: Harper and Row, 1986.

———. *Peace, Love and Healing.* New York: Harper and Row, 1989.

Simonton, O. Carl, and Reid Henson, and Brenda Hampton. *The Healing Journey.* New York and Toronto: Bantam Books, 1992.

Simonton, O. Carl, Stephanie Matthews-Simonton, and James L. Creighton. *Getting Well Again: A Step-by-Step Self-Help Guide to Overcoming Cancer for Patients and Their Families.* New York: Bantam, 1980.

Simonton, Stephanie Matthews, with Robert L. Shook. *The Healing Family.* Toronto and New York: Bantam Books, 1984.

Simpson, Elizabeth Léone. *Notes on an Emergency: A Journal of Recovery.* New York: W. W. Norton and Company, 1982.

Slack, Paul. "Mirrors of Health and Treasures of Poor Men: The Uses of the Vernacular Medical Literature of Tudor England." In *Medicine and Mortality in the 16th Century,* edited by Charles Webster. Cambridge, England: Cambridge University Press, 1979.

Snow, Lois Wheeler. *A Death with Dignity: When the Chinese Came.* New York: Random House, 1974.

Snyder, Marilyn. *An Informed Decision: Understanding Breast Reconstruction.* New York: M. Evans and Company, 1984.

Soiffer, Bill. *Life in the Shadow: Living with Cancer.* San Francisco, Calif.: Chronicle Books, 1991.

Sontag, Susan. *Illness as Metaphor.* New York: Vintage, 1979.

———. *AIDS and Its Metaphors.* New York: Farrar, Straus and Giroux, 1988.

Spacks, Patricia Meyer. *Imagining a Self: Autobiography and Novel in Eighteenth-Century England.* Cambridge, England: Cambridge University Press, 1976.

Sprinker, Michael. "Fictions of the Self: The End of Autobiography." In *Autobiography*, edited by Olney (which see), 321–42.

Starr, George A. *Defoe and Spiritual Autobiography.* Princeton, N.J.: Princeton University Press, 1965.

Stone, Albert E. *Autobiographical Occasions and Original Acts: Versions of American Identity from Henry Adams to Nate Shaw.* Philadelphia: University of Pennsylvania Press, 1982.

Stone, John. *In All This Rain.* Baton Rouge: Louisiana State University Press, 1980.

———. *Renaming the Streets.* Baton Rouge: Louisiana State University Press, 1985.

———. *The Smell of Matches.* Baton Rouge: Louisiana State University Press, 1988.

———. *In the Country of Hearts.* New York: Delacorte, 1990.

Susko, Michael A., ed. *Cry of the Invisible.* Baltimore, Md.: Conservatory Press, 1991.

Tate, David A. *Health, Hope, and Healing.* New York: M. Evans and Company, 1989.

Taylor, Jeremy. *The Rule and Exercises of Holy Dying.* London, England: W. Pickering, 1850.

Teegarden, David, "Holistic Health and Medicine in the 1980s." In *The New Holistic Health Handbook,* edited by Bliss (which see), 14.

Temoshok, Lydia, and Henry Dreher. *The Type C Connection: Bahavioral Links to Cancer and Your Health.* New York: Random House, 1992.

Thompson, Francesca Morosani. *Going for the Cure.* New York: St. Martin's Press, 1989.

Tindall, William York. *John Bunyan, Mechanick Preacher.* New York: Columbia University Press, 1934.

Tolkein, J. R. R. "The Monsters and the Critics." In *An Anthology of Beowulf Criticism,* edited by Louis E. Nicholson, 51–103. Notre Dame, Ind.: University of Notre Dame Press, 1963.

Trapnel, Anna. *A Legacy for Saints, Being Several Experiences of the Dealings of God with Anna Trapnel, in and after Her Conversion.* London, England, 1654.

Turner, Victor W. *The Ritual Process.* Chicago, Ill.: Aldine Publishing Company, 1969.

Tylor, Edward Burnett. *The Origins of Culture.* New York: Harper and Row, 1958.

Ulrich, Betty Garton. *Rooted in the Sky: A Faith to Cope with Cancer.* Valley Forge, Pa.: Judson Press, 1989.

Veatch, Robert M. *Death, Dying, and the Biological Revolution.* New Haven, Conn.: Yale University Press, 1976.

Walton, Izaak. "The Life of Dr. John Donne." In *Lives of Donne and Herbert,* edited by S. C. Roberts. Cambridge, England: Cambridge University Press, 1957.

Webster, Barbara D. *All of a Piece: A Life with Multiple Sclerosis.* Baltimore, Md.: Johns Hopkins University Press, 1989.

Wecksler, Becky Lynn, and Michael Wecksler. *In God's Hand: One Woman's Experience with Breast Cancer.* Scottdale, Pa.: Herald Press, 1989.

Wertenbaker, Lael Tucker. *Death of a Man.* New York: Random House, 1957. Reprint. Boston, Mass.: Beacon Press, 1974.

Wheelwright, Philip. *The Burning Fountain: A Study in the Language of Symbolism.* Bloomington: Indiana University Press, 1954.

Widome, Allen. *The Doctor/the Patient: The Personal Journey of a Physician with Cancer.* Miami, Fla.: Editech Press, 1989.

Wilber, Ken. *Grace and Grit: Spirituality in the Life and Death of Treya Killam Wilber.* Boston and London: Shambhala, 1991.

Williams, Terry Tempest. *Refuge: An Unnatural History of Family and Place.* New York: Pantheon, 1991.